The Wrinkle Cleanse

Also by Cherie Calbom

The Juice Lady's Guide to Juicing for Health

Juicing for Life

The Coconut Diet

The Complete Cancer Cleanse

The Ultimate Smoothie Book

The Wrinkle Cleanse

4 SIMPLE STEPS TO SOFTER, YOUNGER-LOOKING SKIN

• • •

Cherie Calbom, M.S.

Avery

a member of Penguin Group (USA) Inc.

New York   2005

Published by the Penguin Group
Penguin Group (USA) Inc., 375 Hudson Street, New York, New York 10014, USA •
Penguin Group (Canada), 90 Eglinton Avenue East, Suite 700, Toronto, Ontario M4P 2Y3, Canada
(a division of Pearson Penguin Canada Inc.) • Penguin Books Ltd, 80 Strand, London
WC2R 0RL, England • Penguin Ireland, 25 St Stephen's Green, Dublin 2, Ireland (a division of Penguin
Books Ltd) • Penguin Group (Australia), 250 Camberwell Road, Victoria 3124, Australia (a division of
Pearson Australia Group Pty Ltd) • Penguin Books India Pvt Ltd, 11 Community Centre,
Panchsheel Park, New Delhi–110 017, India • Penguin Group (NZ), Cnr Airborne and
Rosedale Roads, Albany, Auckland 1310, New Zealand (a division of Pearson
New Zealand Ltd) • Penguin Books (South Africa) (Pty) Ltd, 24 Sturdee Avenue,
Rosebank, Johannesburg 2196, South Africa • Penguin Books Ltd,
Registered Offices: 80 Strand, London WC2R 0RL, England

First trade paperback edition 2006

The Library of Congress cataloged the hardcover edition as follows:

Calbom, Cherie.
The wrinkle cleanse : 4 simple steps to softer, younger-looking skin / Cherie Calbom.
p.   cm.
Includes bibliographical references and index.
ISBN 1-58333-223-5
1. Skin—Wrinkles.   2. Skin—Care and hygiene.   I. Title.
RL87C35   2005   2004055435
646.7'26—dc22

ISBN 1-58333-255-3 (paperback edition)

Printed in the United States of America
1   3   5   7   9   10   8   6   4   2

Book design by Meighan Cavanaugh

This book is dedicated to every heart
that longs to stay forever young.

～～～～

Contents

~~~~~

Introduction

Do you ever look in the mirror and wonder, Who is that person looking back? Perhaps the years have not been good to your face. Or, maybe there's a new line or two that's just shown up, which concerns you. Whether you're experiencing the first lines of aging or you have many lines, creases, wrinkles, and sags you'd like to erase, you can take action and reclaim your face. I did. And I'm excited to tell you— this program works!

There are a number of steps you can take to slow down or reverse wrinkles and other aspects of aging, including cleansing your body and making wise choices about what you eat and drink, what you think, and how you respond to life's events. This book shows you how to put the dietary and cleansing programs into action to help soften or erase lines, sags, and wrinkles. The principle is simple—get rid of the substances that contribute to wrinkles and add an abundance of life-giving foods that aid the body in "rolling back the years."

The Wrinkle Cleanse program offers four easy steps to help you transform your entire body:

- Step 1, the Quick Cleanses, begins with an all-day vegetable juice fast or a two-day raw-food rejuvenator, both of which will enliven your body and help repair damaged cells.
- Step 2 introduces a low carbohydrate 14-day diet, which includes plenty of vegetables, sprouts, vegetable juices, low-sugar fruit, whole grains, legumes, and lean proteins, and eliminates the substances that increase inflammation and contribute to wrinkles.
- Step 3 outlines the Cleansing Boost programs that will give you an opportunity to experience deep cleansing in the organs of your body, such as your intestinal tract, liver, gallbladder, and kidneys. These unique cleansing programs help to flush away toxins that promote aging and can totally transform your face and your health.
- Step 4 describes the vitamins and minerals that fight aging, and this step can be incorporated into all the other steps of the Wrinkle Cleanse program.

As you follow the four-step program in this book, you can look younger and become healthier. And it's not that hard. These simple steps can produce great results. You may be surprised with the outcome. A number of people following the Wrinkle Cleanse have reported they not only look younger—they've lost weight and overcome a few health challenges, too! The Wrinkle Cleanse four-step program can help you achieve a more youthful appearance and create the excellent health you may have only dreamed about.

During a recent trip, I looked closely at the faces of people passing me in the airport to see how healthy and youthful the average American looked. I was shocked at what I observed. Out of about a hundred people, only a handful looked healthy and had healthful appearing skin. Most had poor coloring, poor skin tone, and a lack of vibrancy. Even quite young people looked rather gray and washed out with reduced skin tone. In short, almost everyone looked like they were aging before their time.

I pondered why so many people had a grayish pallor. I concluded that it's probably the same reason farm-raised salmon have gray-looking flesh and red dye has to be added to make them look palatable. And it's no doubt the same reason the fox that often sits at a neighbor's house by the road I walk in the morning is looking more washed out month by month. The neighbors feed the fox white-bread sandwiches and other processed foods and the farm-raised salmon are fed a processed-food diet, not their customary marine foods. The salmon and the fox, like the people, are not getting a life-giving diet. The manufactured foods they eat are contributing to an appearance that lacks vibrancy and a body that is not healthy. Many people find themselves aging prematurely without any hope of what to do to look younger and more vibrant or to reverse damage to their skin or improve their health.

You may have nearly given up on looking younger. Or maybe you just noticed the first line or two appearing on your face, which sent you into a state of panic and in search of an answer. Wherever you are, no matter what your needs, you will be pleased to know that the Wrinkle Cleanse program works. The "secret" to looking younger and erasing those nasty little wrinkles is in nourishing your body from within, cleansing away toxins and wastes that cause you to age, and feeding your body the best nutrients—from within to the skin. You're about to discover a few secrets that can help you attain a more youthful appearance and at the same time increase your energy and improve your health.

One of the most amazing features of the skin is its ability to heal and restore itself. The skin continues to function as best it can even with abuses and negligence. Imagine how much more healthful and youthful it could be if it were cared for well from within as well as without. As with anything else, we often don't give the skin much thought until signs of aging appear. When we are young, the skin, and the entire body for that matter, is forgiving—usually it recovers from a host of abuses. But as we approach mid-life, usually somewhere in our mid to late thirties, we begin to show signs of aging—our skin looks dry, cracked, or lined. It starts to sag, bags may appear under our eyes, and it can look more scarred, rough, or discolored. Eyelids start to droop and the chin line begins to sag. We look in the mirror and wonder what happened to our face.

Poor food choices, cigarette and alcohol abuse, overindulgence in sweets and other high-carb foods, salt, processed foods, pesticides, and junk foods all take their toll on our faces. Skin cancer threatens us—one out of three Americans will get some form of skin cancer in their lifetime. Damage to our skin may seem irreparable. But many of these symptoms could be avoided or even reversed with the right plan of action.

The dermis, or lower layer of our skin, is made up of collagen and elastin, protein fibers that look similar to mesh netting. These fibers are woven together like fabric. As inflammation, ultraviolet rays (UVA and UVB), and free radical attacks take their toll on these fibers, the skin starts to show lines, wrinkles, sagging, discoloration, and other signs of aging. And, to make matters worse, as the years roll by, production of these fibers slows down. The good news is that you can help reverse that by boosting collagen and elastin production and protecting these fibers from breaking down in the first place.

Cleansing your body, improving your diet, taking the right nutritional supplements, exercising, and even your attitude will not only protect these fibers from breaking down, they will promote production of collagen and elastin—the skin's underlying structure. Additionally, the steps outlined in the Wrinkle Cleanse program go far beyond facial appearance; they can increase your vibrancy, energy, and inner glow. You can add sparkle to your eyes, shine to your hair, and zest to your life. Best of all, you can improve the most important bottom line—your health.

Regardless of the condition of your skin, overall appearance, or the effects of aging that you've experienced until now, improvements can always be made. The Wrinkle Cleanse is about reversing the signs of aging, improving your energy, and restoring that healthy bloom of youth. As you incorporate the Wrinkle Cleanse into your lifestyle, you can restore your skin tone; diminish wrinkles, lines, and creases; and bring back color and vibrancy to your skin and hair. Best of all, and though it may not be your immediate goal, you can improve your health and help prevent serious diseases in the future.

Congratulations! You're on your way to a vibrant, younger-looking you.

1

What Causes Wrinkles?

Is wrinkled, sagging skin a natural, inevitable process of life or is it the result of environmental and lifestyle factors? Researchers have asked this question for decades. Aging is a natural process, but it is now believed that many of the signs and symptoms of getting older usually involve a number of environmental and lifestyle factors. That's good news in one sense. It means that there are steps you can take to slow down the aging process and improve your appearance and health. You can reverse wrinkles, bags, and sags; tighten your skin; improve your health and vitality; increase your mental capacity; and feel more energetic simply by changing certain aspects of your lifestyle, like your diet, attitude, how regularly you exercise, and how often you cleanse your body.

Healthy, younger-looking skin, an energetic body, and a sharp mind is what you can have when you make the Wrinkle Cleanse your antiaging program. You can watch the wrinkles, lines, and bags melt away as you cleanse your body of toxins and feed it superior antioxidant-rich foods and antiaging nutrients. And the secret to the program's success is the four-step process of the Wrinkle Cleanse.

In the pages that follow, you'll learn what makes cleansing the body (also known as detoxification) a key factor in slowing down aging and reversing wrinkles. Most importantly, you'll experience an antiwrinkle program that works. You're about to embark on an exciting journey to a *new you!*

THE FOUNTAIN OF YOUTH

Oh, that mythical fountain of youth! We've longed to find it since the sixteenth century, when Juan Ponce de León sought the mysterious waters that would cure aging. We joke about this elusive fountain and give it little serious thought. But that magical fountain may not be so magical after all. In reality the "waters of youth" can be viewed as the fluids within our own bodies that carry vital nutrients to its trillions of cells, protecting them from damage, feeding them, and flushing away cellular waste and toxins so that they can excrete waste efficiently, repair damage, and thrive.

In 1912 French physician and biologist Dr. Alexis Carrel of the Rockefeller Institute won a Nobel Prize in medicine for his work on the immortality of the cell. Dr. Carrel experimented with various tissues and organs, keeping them alive in laboratory experiments with pure nutrients and religiously cleansing away wastes. He confirmed his theory on cellular immortality through an experiment where he kept a chicken heart alive for twenty-eight years. This experiment was quite remarkable since chickens normally live eight to fifteen years.

Dr. Carrel's research indicated that aging takes place because minute amounts of poisonous substances build up in the blood and fluids throughout the body. His research led Carrel to conclude: "The cell is immortal. It is merely the fluid in which it floats that degenerates. Renew this fluid at proper intervals, and give the cell nourishment upon which to feed, and so far as we know, the pulsation of life may go on forever." He said that the secret to life is to deliver nutrients to and remove toxins from cells; if for any reason the cells can't get nutrients in or remove toxins, they will die from their own waste products.

For years I have looked at research data on reversing aging and observational studies by doctors and researchers on what has worked to help people look and feel younger. It appears that deterioration of the body is primarily due to toxins, wastes, inflammation, and congestion building up throughout the body, along with a shortage of vital nutrients to feed the cells. Cleanse the organs of elimination (intestinal tract, liver, and kidneys); cleanse the blood, lymph, and other fluids; and supply the body with a high-antioxidant, whole foods diet, and we can significantly retard aging and promote youthful cells, tissues, and organs. This equates to a younger face, body, and mind. And this can be the result of your four-step Wrinkle Cleanse program.

WHERE AGING BEGINS

Before you begin the Wrinkle Cleanse program, it's important to know what environmental and biological factors contribute to aging. Armed with knowledge about the causes, you should be more apt to stick with the Wrinkle Cleanse.

Wrinkled, sagging skin begins with the cell plasma membrane. This membrane is where most cell damage occurs. As the membrane ages, it stiffens and loses its fluidity. When it hardens, water cannot pass through the cell carrying vital nutrients in and removing waste efficiently. Waste products build up, enzyme systems slow down, and DNA replication is impaired. The fluids in the spaces between cells (interstitial spaces) become congested and toxic, like a stagnant marsh. Toxins irritate tissues causing inflammation and eventually poisoning the cells.

For decades, scientists, doctors, and researchers have looked for the major contributing factors to aging cells. At least eight have been identified so far and they are all connected to our diet, lifestyle, environment, stress level, and responses to life's events. These factors include:

* environmental toxins and a toxic, congested internal environment
* free radical attacks on our cells*
* inflammation
* weakened immune system
* sun damage
* stress
* insulin resistance
* sleep disturbances

Usually, it's not just one factor that causes us to look and feel older; rather it is several factors working together that cause us to age. However, addressing one issue often deals with several others. As you correct the underlying contributors to wrinkles, the results will show up on your face, in your level of stamina, your quality of sleep, in a sharper mind, and a greater measure of health.

In the pages that follow, you'll not only learn how these factors contribute to wrinkles and other signs of aging, you'll learn how to correct their negative effects.

---

*Free radicals are reactive, unstable oxygen molecules that have lost an electron and that attack cells, causing damage and injury.

ENVIRONMENTAL TOXINS

Toxins wreak havoc within our bodies. In the broad category of environmental toxins, there are a host of wrinkle-causing substances such as industrial chemicals, pesticides, ionizing radiation, free radicals, food additives, toxic fats, high-sugar foods, refined and processed foods, chemical additives, adulterated foods such as GMOs (genetically modified organisms), and excitotoxins (substances such as aspartame and MSG added to foods and beverages that literally stimulate neurons to death). We are bombarded with toxic, congesting, and damaging substances as never before in history. From the air we breathe, the water we drink, the food we eat, to our modern technology and "creature comforts," we are exposed daily to a host of carcinogenic, congesting, and toxic agents.

In addition to all the external toxins, our bodies produce toxins through normal daily functions, called *endotoxins*. Even under ideal health conditions, we need to eliminate by-products (waste) caused by our own cellular and biochemical activities, the thoughts we think, and the stress of living. Nevertheless, if we ate the purest food, drank the cleanest water, breathed the freshest air, and lived in a totally nontoxic environment, our bodies would still generate toxins and waste that would need to be eliminated. Under normal conditions, our body can process endotoxins and a certain amount of external toxins (exotoxins) without a problem, but when an excessive amount is added to the load, our system becomes overwhelmed. "Toxic soup" accumulates throughout our body, poisoning and damaging cells and contributing to wrinkles, lines, sagging skin, and a host of diseases.

FREE RADICALS

In 1956, Denham Harman, MD, PhD, at the University of Nebraska, outlined the theory of free radical damage and aging. He found that most free radicals come from oxygen molecules that have lost an electron, causing them to be reactive, unstable agents. They dance around cells and tissues stealing electrons from healthy molecules, causing damage, and generating more free radicals (also known as *oxidative stress*). We generate free radicals through the normal process of metabolism, and inhale, absorb, and ingest them as well.

Free radicals come from environmental pollutants; radiation; pesticides; herbicides; fungicides; preservatives; damaged fats; medications; drugs, alcohol, and cigarette smoke; airplane travel; auto exhaust; physical overexertion; overexposure to the sun; charbroiled foods; fluorescent lighting; paint, carpet, and furniture fumes; industrial fumes; antibiotic residues in meats and other animal products; mercury amalgam fillings; PCBs; emotional and mental stress—and on it goes. Free radicals are also produced in greater amounts whenever there is trauma, infection, or inflammation. The accumulation of this free radical production creates a host of cellular waste, which adds to the toxic pool of our body.

Free radicals victimize cells by damaging proteins, lipids, DNA, and cellular membranes. Collagen, a fibrous protein that gives our skin a youthful, supple appearance, is particularly susceptible to free radical damage, as is elastin (fibrous protein that resembles collagen). Damage to collagen and elastin leads to wrinkles, flabby skin, droopy eyelids, and sagging chin lines. Free radicals are also responsible for oxidative damage that contributes to the onset and progression of many chronic conditions associated with oxidative stress.

We definitely want to keep free radicals from getting inside our cells, where they do the most damage. The only thing that stops or neutralizes them is a group of nutrients known as antioxidants, which includes vitamins C and E, carotenoids such as beta- and alpha-carotene, flavonoids, alpha lipoic acid, and glutathione. Antioxidants have an even greater affinity for free radicals than for tissue. When consumed or applied to the body, antioxidants give an electron to a free radical, thereby neutralizing it and ending the cascade of tissue damage. Certain antioxidants such as alpha lipoic acid regenerate other antioxidants such as vitamins C and E after they've lost an electron. This is the balance setup for our rejuvenation, but we have to consume plenty of these nutrients, and literally bathe our cells in them, to prevent free radical attacks and stay ahead of the aging game. (If you'd like to know just what kind of free radical activity is taking place in your body, you can order the Free Radical Monitor—a simple home-monitor urine test that reflects the free radical activity in the body. See Resources, p. 249.)

INFLAMMATION

Inflammation is another primary contributor to aging. Nicholas Perricone, MD, author of *The Wrinkle Cure* and *The Perricone Prescription,* has developed the inflammation-aging theory based on years of research as a dermatologist. He says, "Inflammation is the reason you get wrinkles, why you forget everything from where you left your car keys to your neighbor's first name, why you can be irritable and depressed, and why you lose the healthy bloom of youth."

When cells undergo oxidative stress (free radical attack), substances known as *transcription factors* are activated, says Dr. Perricone. "These substances migrate to the cell's nucleus and attach to the DNA, causing the cell to produce inflammatory substances known as *cytokines,* the killer chemicals of our cells. As a result, other chemicals are produced which digest collagen." Dewy, youthful skin is primarily composed of collagen, and when these collagen-digesting chemicals come along, there is no defense against them (unless the free radicals are intercepted by antioxidants before they reach the cell). As collagen is digested, microscarring occurs, which causes wrinkles.

Levels of inflammation-causing substances generally increase with age. When tissue breakdown occurs, such as with free radical attack, white blood cells are mobilized to "clean up" the debris, creating an in-flammatory response. Our goal is to reduce tissue breakdown and the inflammatory response it stimulates.

Dietary imbalances, processed food, chemicals in our food, nutri-tional deficiencies, food allergies, constant infections such as colds and flu, chemical-laden skin-care products, and emotional or mental stress all contribute to inflammation. Reducing stressors that cause inflam-mation by feeding our body superior antioxidant-rich foods, removing inflammatory compounds from our lifestyle, and cleansing our body regularly can protect and heal our cells, tissues, and organs and prevent inflammation.

A WEAKENED IMMUNE SYSTEM

Have you noticed how your skin looks after you've been ill—more wrinkled, drawn, or sagging? When you get sick, right there before your eyes are the results of inflammation at work digesting your colla-gen and stealing another degree of your youthful bloom. Therefore, it's imperative to keep your immune system strong to fight off the "youth stealers."

Catching one cold or flu bug after another is not only bad for your blood vessels, it's highly damaging for your face. Infections, trauma, and inflammation promote inflammatory responses throughout the body.

Therefore, it is important to boost your immune system with lots of antioxidants such as vitamins C and E, carotenes, selenium, alpha lipoic acid, and glutathione to stay healthy. As you power up your immune cells, they can work hard to kill viruses and bacteria that make you sick in the first place. The Wrinkle Cleanse program offers an abundance of nutrient-rich foods that feed the immune system and removes the foods and substances that weaken it.

Sun Damage

The sun's rays, called ultraviolet A and B (UVA and UVB), actually damage the DNA in the skin's cells. This causes inflammation and also causes the cells to become dysfunctional, which means they don't perform properly. Dysfunctional cells have been shown to produce less elastin and collagen (substances in the skin that make it plump and healthy) and to increase photoaging (increased pigmentation). Abnormal pigmentation can take several forms from hyperpigmentation (dark areas) to irregular pigmentation to hypopigmentation (white spots). There is also a thinning of the top layer of the skin that results from sun damage as well as a reduction in the skin's ability to slough off dead layers.

The skin on the face is particularly susceptible to sun damage—it's just half a millimeter thick, which is one hundred times thinner than the skin on the upper back. The sun greatly increases inflammation in facial skin causing damage such as brown spots (age spots), wrinkles, sagging, and leathery looking skin. It is estimated that as much as 80 percent of the visible signs of aging in some individuals, such as wrinkles, age spots, blotchiness, and sagging skin, may be caused by exposure to UV rays.

In the worst scenario, sun damage can lead to skin cancer, which is on the rise. In fact, one in three Americans will get some form of skin cancer in their lifetime. Repeated sunburns are now recognized as a major risk factor for melanoma, the most deadly form of skin cancer. Many people report suffering sunburn while doing something other than lying in the sun, such as walking the dog, reading the paper in the backyard, sitting at an outside café, or gardening. Those most at risk for skin cancer have fair skin and red or blond hair and light-colored eyes; sunburn easily; have numerous moles, freckles, or birthmarks; and have family members with skin cancer.

Tanning booths are not any safer than lying on the beach. They are often marketed as using "harmless" UVA rays, but both UVA and UVB rays damage the skin. UVA rays take longer to damage the skin, but they go deeper into the skin than UVB.

It is advisable to do everything you can to protect your skin from the sun's damaging rays. Here's what you can do:

- Avoid intense sun, especially from 11 a.m. to 3 p.m. when the sun's rays are the strongest
- Don't use tanning booths or sunlamps
- Wear clothing with a tight weave and sun hats during the most intense sun
- Use sunscreen with a sun protection factor (SPF) of 15 or more

The Best Sunscreen and Skin Protector Ingredients

Look for sunscreen that has a minimum SPF of 15, but also choose sunscreen without a lot of chemicals. The skin absorbs what you put on it so it is important to read sunscreen labels. Avoid stuff with lots of words you can't pronounce. Look in health food stores for natural sunscreens that aren't loaded with a lot of chemicals and are based on ingredients that can nourish your skin as well as protect it.

Choose the best ingredients that truly protect and feed your skin:

- *Zinc:* A natural skin healer, zinc is also known to absorb solar radiation.
- *Vitamin C:* Vitamin C is a powerful antioxidant, which neutralizes toxic by-products created in the skin when exposed to the sun. Topical vitamin C works best in the form of freshly activated L-ascorbic acid.
- *Vitamin E:* Protects the skin from photoaging.
- *Green tea extract:* One of the most powerful antioxidants is green tea extract; it has been shown in studies to inhibit the growth of cancerous cells, according to the American Academy of Dermatology.
- *Hyaluronic acid:* Found naturally in the skin, it is known to moisturize and reduce wrinkles.
- *Grape seed extract:* Helps protect the skin against melanoma.

Prevent Sun Damage from Within

When it comes to preventing skin cancer, we're told to slather on the sunscreen and hide under a shade tree or a giant sun hat. But since the invention of sunscreen and all our attempts to hide from the sun, skin cancer rates have gone up, not down.

One of the best ways to prevent sun-damaged skin is to get plenty of carotenes and vitamin C in our diet for skin protection, along with periodic cleansing of the body. Beta-carotene has received the most attention as a protector against sun damage, but alpha-carotene is now believed to be even more powerful in protecting our skin cells from free radical damage caused by the sun. It is known as nature's own sun blocker. And, it appears to be particularly effective in defending against melanomas. The best sources of alpha-carotene include: carrots, pumpkin, chlorella (algae), winter squash, wheatgrass, and yellow, orange, and red bell peppers. Drinking juices made from lots of brightly colored vegetables (with a little low-sugar fruit for flavor, if desired) provides a concentrated form of carotenes to protect the skin.

To avoid brown spots (also known as age spots), get more selenium in your diet. Some of the richest sources of selenium include seafood, Brazil nuts, whole grains, red Swiss chard, lamb, turnips, garlic, eggs, mushrooms, and chicken. Also, steer clear of sugar and other simple carbs along with refined salt (sodium chloride—table salt); these have a browning effect, causing everything from freckles to large brown spots. And, avoid polyunsaturated oils; they tend to turn rancid easily and are oxidized readily in the body creating more free radicals that attack the fat in the skin (known as lipid peroxidation). Use virgin coconut oil for cooking because it is one of the most durable oils (less chance of oxidizing) when it comes to heat and cooking. Use extra virgin, cold-pressed olive oil for salad dressings and light sautéing, if desired. Macadamia nut oil is also acceptable for food preparation, but is not very easy to find. A little expeller-pressed sesame or peanut oil can also be used, but avoid all other unsaturated oils.

Cleansing the body is also very important to prevent sun damage. Brown spots are also called liver spots for good reason. A congested liver can contribute to this kind of skin discoloration along with unsightly little red bumps and spots. Periodic liver cleanses are very helpful to keep your liver clean and functioning well. (See p. 140 for the liver cleanse.) It's a bit like changing the oil and filter in your car. I'll bet you can't imagine not changing your car's oil and filter. But your body is more important to protect than your car, especially since you can't buy a new one. Make liver cleansing a part of your schedule at least twice a year.

Research indicates that *lipid peroxidation* (fat damage) is accelerated at higher elevations. If you live at a high elevation, be particularly careful when going out in the sun and take extra vitamin E (make sure it's the right E with tocotrienols; see Chapter 7 for more information on vitamin E). When we moved to Santa Fe, New Mexico (elevation 7,000 feet above sea level), I sat out in the sun one afternoon for about an hour. Soon afterward, I noticed little brown spots showing up all over my right hand for the first time in my life. My research led me to the information on high elevation and the acceleration of lipid peroxidation and indicated that a greater accumulation of lipofuscin (accumulation of brown pigment in the outer layer of the skin) occurs at higher elevations, especially when there's vitamin E deficiency. So if you live a few thousand feet above sea level, make doubly sure you eat a high-antioxidant diet, supplement with extra vitamins C and E and selenium, and use a good (low chemical) sunscreen with a minimum SPF 15 when you're in the sun, and avoid the most intense hours between 11 a.m. and 3 p.m.

The Skin-Protecting Power of Wheatgrass and Carrot Juice

To avoid sun damage and skin cancer, you need to get an abundance of antioxidants. You can drink an antioxidant-rich shot of "health insurance" every day. Wheatgrass juice is especially rich in the antioxidants alpha- and beta-carotene. You can find wheatgrass juice by the shot glass at most juice bars or you can get a wheatgrass juicer and buy flats of wheatgrass at your local whole foods market and make your own.

Carrot juice is another excellent source of carotenes, rich in both alpha- and beta-carotene. It's great mixed with beet, celery, parsley, spinach, and a little bit of lemon or apple juice for flavor, which will give you even more carotenes. I like to add ginger root, too, because it has anti-inflammatory properties and is rich in zinc, plus it really spices up the juice. I add lemon for vitamin C and bioflavonoids because it adds a fresh citrus flavor. (Vitamin C is very protective of the skin when it comes to sun damage.)

Benefits of the Sun

Despite the danger, we still need about thirty minutes of sunshine on our skin almost every day to prevent everything from seasonal affective disorder, to breast and colon cancer, and a deficiency of vitamin D, which can cause rickets. Granted, we don't want to sunburn, but neither do we want to stay completely away from our best source of vitamin D.

When you do get a bit of sunshine, choose the cooler, early morning hours before 11 a.m. or late afternoon after 3 p.m. and follow the instructions for preventing sunburn with a good sunscreen and lots of carotenes in your diet. With this plan of action, you can get your thirty-minute daily dose of vitamin D responsibly. As you follow the guidelines for skin protection, you can wisely prevent sun damage while responsibly taking advantage of the sun.

This plan makes more sense than just hiding in the shade for the rest of your life and slathering blobs of chemicals all over your skin just to walk down the street. You can soak up your vitamin D from the sun a few minutes each day, if you do so wisely by including the best dietary supplements and topical applications that protect your skin from damage.

STRESS

There's nothing like stress lines on the face to make us look older. Stress is the mental, emotional, or physical strain caused by such things as anxiety, abuse, or overwork. Stress has been shown to increase cortisol (a hormone that is produced by the adrenal glands). When there is a stressor, whether it is viral, environmental, physical, behavioral, or psychological, a complex series of actions takes place in the endocrine system, resulting in increased adrenal hormone release. Chronically elevated cortisol is harmful in many respects—it adversely affects the heart, brain cells are at risk for damage, blood sugar rises, the immune system is depressed, making us more susceptible to infections, and we gain weight, particularly around the midsection.

Stress also elevates prolactin (a hormone produced in the pituitary gland that stimulates progesterone) and TSH (thyroid-stimulating hormone). It can increase catecholamines (organic compounds that affect the sympathetic nervous system) and corticosteroids (steroid hormones produced by the adrenal gland—involved in metabolism and the immune system), and it mobilizes tissue calcium. All these endocrine changes are a setup for physical problems and premature aging.

Long-term stress also has been associated with conversion of protein to carbohydrates and fat, which results in weight gain, increased LDL (bad cholesterol), reduced HDL (good cholesterol), increased platelet count, and a lowered stimulation threshold in the brain.

When it comes to wrinkles, stress is a major contributing factor. Lines tend to form around the eyes, furrows show up between the brows, and creases develop around the lips. Along with the obvious changes in facial expression due to inner turmoil, the cause of these facial changes can also be attributed to a depletion of vitamin C, which is used up in greater measure when we're under stress. Vitamin C, which is depleted when we're stressed, is essential for production of collagen, which supports the skin and gives it firmness. As a result, we become susceptible to loss of facial tone—the skin starts to sag, becomes flabby, and lines increase.

Vitamin C is a cofactor for several enzymes that are involved in the synthesis of carnitine. As levels of vitamin C diminish, carnitine levels drop, making it difficult for cells to oxidize fats and create energy. Consequently, we feel and look more tired.

Stress caused by life's events, which is what most of us experience, is not necessarily bad. It is our response to the stressors that can be either positive or negative. As we learn to deal with stress in a positive way, we can prevent the cascade of negative reactions it could otherwise produce within the body.

To combat the negative effects of stress, take a few actions each day to de-stress. Here's what you can do:

- Take a walk and breathe deeply
- Make a cup of herbal tea and sip it slowly as you take time out to relax
- Take a fifteen-minute work break during which you think and discuss only positive thoughts
- Take a bath at the end of the day by candlelight and relaxing music
- Set aside ten minutes to meditate or pray
- Make time to talk with someone you find very encouraging
- Get a massage or a facial on a day off from work
- Schedule times to get away—just for you—like a weekend at your favorite lake, mountain, beach, or spa
- At least once a year, take a health vacation someplace that offers a raw-food and juice-cleansing program along with lots of pampering such as massages and facials and time to rest

Smile Often, Think Young, Love Well

Smile—you might start looking younger. The healing, rejuvenating power of a smile can do wonders to reduce stress and heal the body. A Russian researcher investigated a monastery that was having remarkable results with patients with all forms of degenerative diseases. Part of the therapy employed at the monastery was smiling. Each participant was required to stand erect at all times and wear a smile. A smile is a physical manifestation of contentment and joy. The act of putting a smile on your face registers in the hypothalamus where endorphins (the feel-good chemicals) are produced, and sends a signal that "all is well." Try it. Smile. Hold that smile for ten seconds and see how you feel.

If you smile enough you begin to experience joy. And joy leads to contentment, even in the most stressful situations. Trust, peace of mind, choosing not to hurry or worry, and joy are antidotes to stress. The Bible's Proverbs says that a merry heart is good medicine.

When we create new actions that are positive, our body gets the message and starts to act on the signals we send. When we smile, the brain picks it up and sends messages throughout the body that everything is going well. Then no matter what the situation, from traffic jams to an out-of-sorts boss, we can sail through the situation unaffected by external circumstances.

Think Young

Have you ever noticed how some people in their golden years just seem perennially young? I had an aunt who was young in spirit until the day she died at ninety-four. She was never old—always ready to go somewhere, see something different, or learn something new. She was an inspiration to everyone who knew her. That spirit showed up on her face; she always had beautiful skin with few wrinkles.

You can choose to think young and keep that youthful spirit of wonderment, hope, adventure, and enjoyment of life. Look around you as often as you can, whether on a walk in your neighborhood or into the face of a friend, and choose to appreciate the gift you see. Enjoying life's small gifts is a choice we can make each day that pays huge dividends.

Love Well

Family support and a close social network are important factors in staying young. Deepak Chopra summarizes this well in *Grow Younger, Live Longer,* "For the benefit of your physical, emotional, and spiritual well-being, generate more love in your life. When you make love the most important thing in your life, your mind and body resonate with timelessness."

Love is a choice. You can choose to love well. Loving without reservation benefits you and the ones you love. And you can choose to love life also and participate in it fully. Why not love and live life to the fullest? What have you got to lose other than a few lines on your face? Health educator Stephen Cherniske says: "Approach anti-aging not from a fear of death, but from a love of life."

INSULIN RESISTANCE

There is growing evidence from centenarian studies around the world that balanced, healthy insulin levels are clear markers for longevity. Researchers are finding from these studies that centenarians have one thing in common—they all have relatively low sugar and triglycerides for their age.

Maintaining cells that are sensitive to insulin and thereby preventing insulin resistance is another key factor in preventing wrinkles. When cells are not sensitive to insulin, levels of this hormone go up and it accumulates in the blood. This condition is known as insulin resistance and it is generally recognized to be a major contributor to aging and age-related chronic diseases.

When the body notices that blood sugar has elevated, it releases insulin to shuttle the sugar off to storage units known as adipose tissue (fat cells) where it gets stored in the form of glycogen. Once glycogen stores are filled up, the excess sugar is stored as saturated fat.

When we think of insulin, we most often think of its relationship to blood sugar. But one of the primary roles of insulin is pushing glucose out of the blood and into muscle where it is converted into energy. It is also responsible for storage of nutrients—insulin stores nutrients such as magnesium in cells. If cells become insulin resistant, they will become magnesium deficient as well as deficient in many other important nutrients.

Also, when our blood sugar levels go up, glucose will compete with vitamin C for entry into cells. Vitamin C is needed by white blood cells to keep them strong and healthy so they can attack and destroy bacteria, viruses, and cancer cells—a process known as *phagocytosis*. Our bodies can't manufacture vitamin C; we have to ingest it and accumulate it in our cells. The more glucose in our bloodstream, the less vitamin C will enter the immune cells because glucose has a tendency to beat out vitamin C in uptake. It doesn't take a lot of glucose to experience this effect. A blood sugar level of 120 reduces the phagocytic index 75 percent; a healthy blood sugar level should be between 60 and 100 mg. (The phagocytic index is the rate at which white blood cells gobble up bacteria, viruses, and cancer cells.) The more sugar in our bloodstream, the more we'll be susceptible to bacterial or viral infections and cancer, and the more inflammation we'll experience in the body, which causes us to age prematurely.

Eating sugar, or foods that easily convert to sugar in the body, whether sweets, alcohol, refined flour products like pasta and rolls, or white potatoes or white rice (all high on the glycemic index) causes blood sugar levels to rise. Eating high-carbohydrate foods, especially the refined carbs, causes the pancreas to secrete extra insulin and usually too much of this hormone is pumped out at any given time. Then we experience spikes and dips in blood sugar levels. This yo-yo effect can lead to insulin resistance. At this point we can say we've entered the fast track of aging. As you can see, it is very important to stabilize your blood sugar levels and keep them stable as much as possible by keeping these foods to a minimum or completely excluding them from the diet. (If you suspect that you may be insulin resistant, take the Insulin Resistance Quiz found on p. 232.)

SLEEP DISTURBANCES

It's no mistake that sleep has been called a fabulous beautifier, as in "get your beauty sleep." Sleep restores cognition and immunity and rejuvenates us emotionally and hormonally; our faces look rested and our eyes sparkle with life. When we sleep well, our body is able to repair cells and release healing hormones. But, depriving ourselves of adequate sleep accelerates the aging process. It can also lead to heart disease, stroke, cancer, diabetes, and obesity.

Sleep deprivation decreases the body's production of growth hormone (GH), an important fat burner and muscle builder, and accelerates fat gain. Growth hormone levels decrease as we age, beginning their decline around the age of thirty-five. Signs of GH deficiency include weight gain around the abdomen, less energy and vitality, lowered self-esteem, diminished health, decreased HDL (good cholesterol), and an increase in LDL (bad cholesterol). L-glutamine (an amino acid) releases GH from the pituitary gland. Sweets and other foods high on the glycemic index (high-carb foods) that may not even taste sweet, like white potatoes or refined-flour bread, turn the GH releasing mechanism off, which is mostly released while we sleep. In addition, when we are sleep-deprived, levels of leptin, a hormone that regulates food cravings, drop and we usually crave fats and carbohydrates, especially sweets. While these foods should not be consumed as a part of the Wrinkle Cleanse Diet, you should especially avoid them in the evening no matter what the event or situation if you want a good night's sleep.

Melatonin is another hormone produced during the dark hours by the pineal gland in the brain; it prepares our body to fall asleep naturally. Melatonin also helps quench the corrosive free radical hydroxyl. Since the brain is made up of a large amount of fat, it is prone to free radical attacks, so we need to make sure it is protected with plenty of deep, restful sleep during which melatonin is produced. Melatonin may also be responsible for many cleansing activities while we're asleep that reverse the action of toxins created during various stresses and illnesses. A lack of sleep can cause an accumulation of these toxic substances that lead to the formation of wrinkles and age spots due to fat damage.

Powerful healing hormones are released as we sleep. Much of the work of repair and restoration is accomplished during the night. Many experts specify that some of the most important work is done between 10 p.m. and midnight. It is important not to eat after 7:30 p.m. so that your body is not engaged in digestion when you are trying to go to sleep and when your body should be in the detoxification mode. Eating a large meal at night can interrupt the sleep cycle because the body has to concentrate on digesting all that food. This makes us restless and interferes with the body's restorative work.

Getting a Good Night's Sleep

The more you move away from your normal sleep cycle, the faster you age. To gain the most from rejuvenating sleep, it's important to go to bed between 9:30 and 10 p.m. most evenings and get eight to eight and a half hours of sleep each night.

If you have trouble falling asleep, begin to quiet your mind an hour before you want to fall asleep. Anxious thoughts can keep you up half the night. Make a conscious decision to trust in God or your Higher Power to help you handle the situation causing anxiety and choose to let go of thinking about it at night. Take a warm bath, read something relaxing or inspiring, drink a cup of chamomile tea, play soothing music, or do whatever else works for you to relax. Refrain from anything that raises your blood pressure, such as arguments or watching TV. Herbs such as valerian root can be helpful. There are supplements that combine valerian root with other sleep-enhancing herbs that can help you sleep more restfully. (See Resources, p. 251.) Melatonin can be helpful if your body is not producing enough on its own. However, taking melatonin over a long period of time can cause the pineal glad to become less active. Therefore, the dosage should be small—1 g or less, and should not be taken every day. It is best to reserve melatonin for travel, especially when changing time zones, or when you are experiencing anxiety, stress, or insomnia. If you have habitual problems with sleep, consider working on your thyroid health.

Your Thyroid Gland

An underactive thyroid gland is often a cause of sleep problems as well as weight gain and premature aging. Many people who have an underactive thyroid can sleep for the first few hours of the night and then are restless for the remainder. When the thyroid gland gets starved and dysfunctional, full-blown insomnia is not unusual, and that can definitely contribute to looking older and more tired. Thyroid tests are not sensitive enough to identify a thyroid that needs nutritional help. For this reason, many people suffer from an undernourished thyroid gland and are unaware that numerous symptoms such as fatigue, weight gain, forgetfulness, nail problems, hair loss, and cold hands and feet are the result of a starved thyroid.

It is important to feed the thyroid what it needs and to avoid foods that cause the gland stress. Iodine-rich foods that nourish the thyroid include: seafood, fish, eggs, cranberries, and sea vegetables. (You may also benefit from kelp tablets or iodine drops.) Foods that tax the thyroid include: alcohol, sugars, refined grains, hydrogenated and partially hydrogenated fats (transfatty acids), and caffeine (coffee, black tea, sodas, chocolate). Many foods are iodine blockers (known as goitrogens), and should also be avoided, including soy foods and soy oil, peanuts and peanut oil, turnips, cabbage, mustard, pine nuts, and millet.

You should also treat Candida albicans (yeast infections) and work on emotional stress (anger, grief, fear, worry, guilt), environmental stress (toxic chemicals), and avoid pesticides, mercury, fluoride, and pollutants. Avoid excessive exercise (moderate exercise is good for the thyroid; excessive is not), and a number of medical treatments (various medications, radiation, X-rays). If you suspect that you may have low thyroid, take the quiz on page 240.

THE KEY TO ERASING WRINKLES

All these factors contribute to the body's toxic load and to the aging process. But you're not stuck with their results. The Wrinkle Cleanse shows you how to cleanse the body and reverse the damaging effects of toxins and a wrinkle-causing lifestyle. With this program, you can achieve a more youthful appearance, softer skin, and a healthier body in a relatively short time. It's not that hard. Small efforts can produce huge benefits.

Changing some simple lifestyle practices and scheduling periodic detoxification days is key to erasing wrinkles and lines, and eliminating sags, bags, discoloration, sun damage, and even disease. The four-step Wrinkle Cleanse program is key to rejuvenating your body and mind. It will help you reverse unfavorable internal conditions by cleansing your body and ridding it of toxins that cause premature aging.

By eating an abundance of life-giving, revitalizing whole foods, increasing your consumption of antioxidants, cleansing the body of toxins periodically, fasting occasionally, getting adequate rest and sleep, scheduling a cleansing (detox) week at least once a year at a health institute or spa, making time for regular exercise, practicing emotional balance and stress reduction, and developing spiritual practices that produce well-being, you can reverse the internal conditions that cause premature aging and rejuvenate your body, soul, and spirit.

Keys to Antiaging

Eat an abundance of life-giving, revitalizing whole foods

Increase your consumption of antioxidants

Strengthen your immune system

Balance your blood sugar levels and prevent insulin resistance

Cleanse your body periodically

Fast occasionally

Schedule a detox week at least once a year at a cleansing health institute or spa

Get eight to eight and a half hours of sleep a night and adequate rest and relaxation

Make time for regular exercise

Practice emotional balance and stress reduction

Develop spiritual well-being

As you put these practices into action, you can reverse the internal conditions that cause premature aging and prevent serious diseases in the future. *The Wrinkle Cleanse* will help you implement all of these antiaging lifestyle practices into four easy steps. This plan of action will create a healthy internal state that encourages well-nourished, supple cells. This is the ultimate antiaging program. It goes far beyond just topical antiwrinkle applications—which I'm all for—and addresses the internal causes of aging. Armed with this knowledge and the action steps in *The Wrinkle Cleanse,* your new youthful appearance and healthy, vibrant looks can become the topic of conversation. To reclaim your face, actually your whole life, it's time to take action *now.*

But before you start your renewal program, Chapter 2 will explain why you should eat the wrinkle cleanse foods encouraged in the Wrinkle Cleanse Diet. You'll discover how profoundly the food you eat effects how you look and can help you look younger than your years.

2

The Wrinkle Cleanse Foods

The skin doesn't lie. We are what we eat when it comes to our faces as well as our health. Research tells us that eating the right foods can have a significant effect on how young we look. The Wrinkle Cleanse Diet offers an abundance of revitalizing whole foods that help us look younger. They're rich in antioxidants (the wrinkle fighters!) and other nutrients that fight inflammation, balance blood sugar, support the immune system, and strengthen collagen and elastin.

Choosing the diet that's best for you can be a bit like putting together a puzzle of carbs, fat, and protein. In the beginning it's a bit confusing, but as the pieces fall into place, a picture emerges—the diet that is healthiest in a form you can readily incorporate. The results will be a program that can optimize your body's ability to ward off disease and slow down signs of aging.

Planning a Wrinkle Cleanse diet is easy. It involves simple and wise carbohydrate, fat, and protein choices that will help you formulate a healthy diet for every day, even when you're on the go with a very busy lifestyle. Following are the food recommendations that will help you begin turning back the hands of time.

The Mediterranean Diet: A Foundation of Health

A scientific study published in the *Journal of the American College of Nutrition* (2001) titled "Skin Wrinkling: Can Food Make a Difference?" supports the belief that diet has a significant impact when it comes to antiaging. This population study evaluated the diet and sunlight damage of 177 people (Greeks, Australians, and Swedes). The results of the study indicated that skin damage was associated *least* with people who ate more vegetables, olive oil, fish, and legumes and who had a low intake of butter, margarine, milk products, meat, and sugary foods. Foods associated with the most skin damage were full-fat milk, red meat, potatoes, soft drinks, cordials, and sweets such as cakes and pastries.

The benefits of a Mediterranean diet (which this program typifies) for wrinkle prevention and antiaging in general shouldn't be too surprising because it has long been associated with longevity and good health. People following the Mediterranean diet have a dramatic decrease in coronary artery disease. The incidence of breast cancer is less than half in the Greek population eating a traditional diet compared to the U.S. population eating a typical Western diet, and total cancer incidence is about 20 percent less.

Greece and Spain are countries where the consumption of vegetables and olive oil are high. The vegetables that make up a significant portion of the Greek diet include wild greens, which contain high amounts of flavonoids (phytochemicals that have powerful antioxidant properties)—

much higher than red wine or tea. The amount of vegetables eaten by Greeks is higher than that of Americans: legume (beans, lentils, split peas) consumption is 30 percent higher, and fish thirteen times higher. The olive oil used liberally in the Mediterranean diet is obtained from the whole olive by means of physical pressure and without the use of chemicals, whereas most vegetable oils in the United States are extracted by solvents (chemicals) and heat.

We can conclude from these studies that one of the very best antiaging "facials" you can give yourself is what you put *inside* your body. You can wrap, scrub, soak, cleanse, moisturize, and peel your face for a lifetime and never achieve the results you can have when you incorporate the Wrinkle Cleanse dietary program with beneficial external treatments.

If you're ready to renew your face, indeed your entire body, start with the kind of whole foods eaten around the Mediterranean. These foods can help you look and feel younger and healthier.

VEGETABLES AND LEGUMES

Most plant foods such as sprouts, legumes, herbs, sea vegetables, and brightly colored vegetables contain an abundance of nutrients, particularly the antioxidants. These foods are powerhouses of vitamins, minerals, enzymes, phytochemicals, and fiber. Even on a carb-restricted diet, we can eat large amounts of most vegetables, salad greens, sea vegetables, and sprouts and never gain weight or feel deprived. The high-fiber content of such foods slows down the rate that sugars enter the bloodstream, thereby lowering insulin secretion. Vegetables, sprouts, herbs, sea vegetables, legumes, and salad greens should be your primary source of carbohydrates on the Wrinkle Cleanse Diet.

These foods offer lots of soluble and insoluble fiber. Insoluble fiber is a polysaccharide that resists digestion by the body's acids and enzymes, and is very important in human nutrition, especially for colon health. Soluble fiber (also important for colon health) such as pectin (found primarily in fruit, seeds, and peels), gums (sticky substance found inside plants), and mucilages (found in plant secretions and seeds), forms a gel-like substance in the intestinal tract that increases bulk and binds to bile acids (which contain cholesterol) in the digestive tract so that it can't be reabsorbed. Fiber, sometimes called nature's broom, helps keep the colon clean and decreases transit time for waste elimination. Fiber is found in fruits, vegetables, whole (unrefined) grains, herbs, sea vegetables, legumes (beans, lentils, split peas), and seeds.

A diet rich in brightly colored vegetables is a diet rich in antioxidants

Organically Grown Food

As often as possible, purchase organically grown vegetables, fruit, grains, nuts, seeds, legumes, and animal products in order to reduce your exposure to pesticides and to increase the nutrient value of your food. Produce that is sprayed with pesticides, fungicides, herbicides, and grown with chemical fertilizers introduces toxins into our bodies that contribute to free radical formation that can contribute to wrinkles and disease.

Plants absorb nutrients from the soil, but they also take up pesticides. Healthy soil is rich in minerals and alive with microorganisms. Pesticides and chemical fertilizers kill these much-needed microorganisms. Chemical fertilizers do not replenish the soil in any manner close to traditional composting and other traditional natural practices that nourish soil.

Chemical fertilizers also generate a high level of nitrogen in soil, which increases the amount of protein in crops, but reduces the quality of the protein. Organically managed soils release nitrogen in smaller amounts over a longer time than conventional fertilizers, creating crops with higher quality protein.

A 2001 study published in the *Journal of Alternative and Complementary Medicine,* stated that on average, organic produce contained 27 percent more vitamin C, 21 percent more iron, and 29 percent more magnesium than conventional produce, and all twenty-one minerals compared in the study were higher in the organic produce. An abundance of antioxidants will help your body neutralize free radicals more effectively and reduce inflammation. You might say organic produce is not only good for your health—it's good for your face.

When organic produce is not available, it's better to eat vegetables that are commercially grown than to omit them. Wash or peel produce to remove any pesticide residue and waxes on skins. There are vegetable washes that can help you remove external pesticides. Unfortunately, systemic pesticides, those that enter the plant's interior, cannot be removed.

like carotenes, vitamins C and E, glutathione, and selenium. These are the nutrients that protect the trillions of cells in our body from the ravages of free radical attack, reduce inflammation, and strengthen the immune system. Choose a variety of colorful vegetables—dark green, orange, yellow, purple, and red—and eat five to six servings each day. Select organically grown produce whenever possible to avoid pesticides, herbicides, and fungicides and increase your nutritional intake.

Often legumes (beans, lentils, and split peas) are simply referred to as beans, but whatever we call them, all three are good plant sources of protein and nutrients. They are low in cost and high in fiber; in fact, these complex carbohydrates are second only to bran in their fiber content. The particular fiber in beans helps modify fatty substances in the blood, which no doubt is one of the reasons beans have been shown in research to lower LDL (bad cholesterol). They also help regulate bowel function.

Lentils are a fair source of iron, and when combined with vitamin C-rich foods such as broccoli, parsley, bell peppers, tomatoes, or dark leafy greens, iron absorption is enhanced. There are many varieties of beans, such as azuki, cannellini, and pink beans. Why not try a new variety? Some beans, such as mung and red lentils, are great sprouted, which increases the B vitamin and vitamin C content that is absent in dried beans. You can enjoy all varieties of legumes on the Wrinkle Cleanse Diet and they are healthiest when grown organically.

Wrinkle Cleanse Vegetables and Legumes

Artichokes

Asparagus

Bamboo shoots

Beans (green and yellow wax, aduki, black, butter, garbanzo, kidney, lentils, lima, and split peas)

Beets and beet greens

Bell peppers (green, red, yellow, purple)

Bok choy

Broccoflower

Broccoli

Broccoli rabe

Broccolini

Brussels sprouts

Cabbage (Chinese, green, red, savoy)

Carrot

Cassava

Cauliflower

Celery

Celeriac

Chard

Chayote

Collards

Cucumber

Dandelion greens

Eggplant

Endive

Fennel

Jicama

Kale

Kohlrabi

Lettuce (all varieties, including romaine, bibb/Boston, iceberg, red leaf, green leaf, spring greens/mesclun)

Mushrooms (all varieties, including portobello, shiitake, oyster, straw, whole button)

Mustard greens

Okra

Onions

Parsley

Peas

Pea pods

Radicchio

Radishes

Rutabaga

Sauerkraut

Scallions

Sorrel

Spinach

Sprouts (all varieties)

Squash (Hubbard, spaghetti, acorn, yellow summer, zucchini)

Tomatillo

Tomato (all varieties, including cherry, Roma, plum, yellow pear, red [includes beefsteak], sun-dried)

Taro root

Turnips

Water chestnuts

Watercress

RAW FOODS

Raw foods will put a sparkle in your eye, add luster to your hair, and a youthful freshness to your skin like nothing else can do. Raw foods are cleansing, rejuvenating, and energizing. Raw fruits and vegetables are the most nutrient-rich foods we can eat, and raw vegetables in particular are among the best antiaging foods on earth. They are loaded with enzymes, vitamins, minerals, fiber, and phytochemicals. As soon as we cook our vegetables, we destroy many of the life-giving nutrients like vitamins and enzymes; therefore, it is important to eat some of our plant-based foods uncooked as often as possible.

A diet rich in raw plant-based foods such as sprouts, herbs, vegetables, fruit, nuts, and seeds will supply the body with an abundance of enzymes, which most of us are very short on these days—cooking and processing destroys them. They are only found in raw food and foods warmed or dehydrated at low temperatures (118°F or below). As we age, our enzyme reserves decrease. Without adequate enzymes to break down the food we eat, more undigested material accumulates in our body, which leads to inflammation, weight gain, poor digestion, fatigue, and wrinkles. Raw foods are replete with enzymes, which aid in digestion and help prevent aging and disease.

Strive to eat some raw plant foods with every meal, such as a salad, sliced tomatoes or avocado, berries in a smoothie or on whole grain cereal, or raw seeds, nuts, or sprouts sprinkled on your favorite salad or cooked dish.

Wrinkle Cleanse Rejuvenation

Several years ago I had a traveling schedule that would have made the Energizer Bunny tired. I was flying about 125,000 miles a year giving presentations for the George Foreman grill on QVC (Philadelphia and Germany) and The Shopping Channel (TSC) of Canada in Toronto. Tired didn't begin to describe how I felt and looked. My eyelids in particular began looking older by the day—droopy, with folds and creases on folds, and smaller, too. I'd look at old pictures and wonder what happened to the much larger eyes I saw in the pictures. Even my husband commented that maybe I should get an eyelift.

I knew that if I was looking a lot older at an accelerated rate, unfavorable things were also happening internally—perhaps setting me up for a major disease. I kicked off my cleansing program with a diet of raw foods and a three-day vegetable juice fast. I faithfully juiced vegetables every day. Following my Wrinkle Cleanse program vigorously, I cut out all simple carbs from my diet, even though I'm a mashed potato lover.

It paid off in short order. I was able to renew my body at the cellular level and it showed up with facial skin tightening. The droops and folds disappeared from my eyelids, my eyes looked larger again, and even my chin line toned up. Someone even asked me if I'd had an eyelift. And my husband began telling me how good I looked. Best of all, I really felt good. Alive! Actually, I felt more alive than I'd felt in years.

RAW VEGETABLE JUICES

Raw juices are "alive" and packed with an abundance of nutrients—from phytochemicals and enzymes to vitamins and minerals. They are rich in enzymes, which greatly benefit the digestive system. They do most of the excellent things that solid raw foods do, but because they are broken down into an easily absorbable form, they put minimum strain on the digestive system. It is believed that the nutrients from fresh juices are at work in the bloodstream within about thirty minutes of our drinking them.

The alkalinity of raw vegetable juices, in particular, is a powerful ally in our fight against aging, since overacidity is an underlying cause of ailments that rob us of our health, vitality, and youthful appearance. The standard American diet (SAD) is dominated by acid-forming foods such as sweets, animal products, alcohol, coffee, and refined grains. Vegetable juices are an excellent way to bring more of an acid-alkaline balance to the system, while at the same time feeding it an abundance of antioxidants.

Ginger Root

Include fresh ginger root as often as possible in fresh vegetable juices and recipes. I juice it nearly every day. It's been shown in scientific studies that ginger root has anti-inflammatory properties and can be very helpful in your fight against inflammation and aging. Ginger is also rich in zinc, an important mineral for strengthening the immune system, healing the skin, thwarting sunburn, and preventing senile purpura (purple spots under the skin caused by bleeding).

Raw vegetable juices can help you cleanse the body of substances that can cause oxidative stress and cellular damage. Our bodies pick up a lot of toxic junk every day—everything from chemicals in packaged and convenience foods to air pollution that pours into our air, water, and soil, and pesticide-sprayed produce. Heavy metals, antibiotics, synthetic hormones, anesthetics, drug residues, pesticides, fungicides, herbicides, industrial chemicals, and solvents all collect within our bodies. Every cell, organ, and system is affected. When the body becomes overwhelmed and can no longer keep up with neutralizing and eliminating this accumulation of toxic stuff, we age much faster than we should. The only way to halt this process is to cleanse the body of these toxins and wastes because all this toxic material doesn't make its way out of the body on its own, if we continue to go about eating as usual.

Lee Bueno-Aguer, author of *Fast Your Way to Health,* has found that when the body is cleansed, the skin becomes beautiful, glowing, youthful in appearance, and has good color. Lines and wrinkles soften or disappear, skin tone evens out, the whites of the eyes become whiter, the eyes sparkle again as they did in youth. She found firsthand that wholesome food and periodic fasts can indeed turn on the fountain of youth within.

Cleansing the body with raw foods and vegetable juices is no doubt the single most potent antidote to aging available anywhere. Known as the famous *Rohsaftkur* (raw juice cure) in Europe, the raw foods and juice-cleansing program has done wonders to reverse aging for countless numbers of people. Leslie and Susannah Kenton, authors of *Raw Energy,* say:

> Standard theories of nutrition have never quite been able to explain why drinking nothing but fresh raw juices for a period varying from two days to several weeks works such miracles, for "miracle" is the word used by many of those who have had the Rohsaft experience. The visible benefits include a lessening in the number and depth of lines on the face, a firming of body contours, and healthier looking nails and hair.

Juicing is the best way I know to get a high concentration of all the beneficial elements found in vegetables to help fight premature aging. Fresh raw juices made from organic vegetables (and a little fruit for flavor, as desired) provide a concentration of the most beneficial nutrients that is far superior to any supplement that we can buy. Fruits and vegetables have the perfect proportions of elements that act synergistically to give our body what it needs. No matter how sophisticated a pill or man-made formula may be, it cannot come close to the balanced perfection of whole foods. Juicing unlocks this power and gives it to us in a concentrated, easily assimilated form. It would be difficult, if not impossible, to eat in a day the amount of vegetables that we can drink in a glass of juice.

A number of years ago juicing got a "bad rap" in the sense that many individuals in the media began telling people that eating vegetables and fruit was the only way to go because juice has no fiber. That thinking simply is not true. Juice has plenty of soluble fiber—pectin, gums, and mucilages—that is very beneficial for the intestinal tract. And juice offers the opportunity to consume produce, and parts of plants such as leaves, stems, seeds, and peels, that we would probably never eat otherwise, along with making it easier for us to consume more servings of vegetables in a day.

I have never recommended that anyone give up eating vegetables and fruit in trade for juice, but rather that we do both. Juice is a marvelous supplement to a high-fiber, whole foods diet that includes the insoluble fiber from vegetables, fruit, legumes, and whole grains. It's also a great way to cleanse the body. Through juice fasting and other cleansing programs that incorporate fresh vegetable juice, we can greatly facilitate the elimination of toxins and waste, restore acid-alkaline balance to our body, and achieve a vibrant healthy glow.

Start your day with an eight- to ten-ounce glass of fresh vegetable juice and you will be providing your body with a cornucopia of cleansing and protective elements that should take you through the morning energized and alert. If the idea of making fresh juice daily seems daunting, it may be encouraging to know that millions of people have found juicing to be as easy as any other daily routine when they have the right juicer—one that's easy to use and clean. If you get a juicer with only a few parts to clean and a good motor (half horsepower), along with a feature that ejects the pulp, you're more likely to incorporate vegetable juicing on a regular basis. If you work outside the home, try preparing your vegetables the night before so that you only need to push them through the juicer in the morning and sip away as you get ready for work. You will find delicious and easy juice recipes in Chapter 8.

I include some vegetables, namely carrots and beets, that some experts say to avoid because they contain more sugar than many other vegetables. But these two vegetables have a high nutrient content and are so rich in antioxidants that they should not be excluded from any antiaging diet. Actually, carrots are in the low glycemic index category, and they're one of the richest sources of alpha- and beta-carotene, which are so very important for skin health. Beets, in the moderate glycemic index category, are rich in carotenes and iron; they are also traditionally recommended for cleansing the liver. I balance these two vegetables with very low-sugar veggies such as cucumber, celery, parsley, spinach, and kale and flavor with lemon and ginger root to make the total juice content relatively low in sugar.

The "Super Hero" Antiwrinkle Juices

Following are the juice ingredients found to be very helpful in fighting wrinkles.

Beet juice has been used traditionally to cleanse and support the liver. It's rich in carotenes, and the leaves, which you can juice, too, along with the stems, have an abundance of minerals, especially iron, magnesium, calcium, manganese, and potassium.

Carrot juice is one of nature's riches sources of alpha- and beta-carotene. (Alpha-carotene is considered nature's best natural sun blocker.)

Cucumber and bell pepper juices are excellent sources of silicon, which is known to improve the appearance of the skin. The pH of the cucumber is close to that of the skin and may help prevent wrinkles. (Green bell pepper also offers some iodine, which is food for the thyroid gland.)

Ginger juice is an excellent anti-inflammatory; it's also rich in zinc.

Green leafy vegetable juices such as parsley (an herb), spinach, kale, chard, beet tops, and mustard greens, along with wheatgrass, are particularly rich in chlorophyll, antioxidants, and alkalizing minerals.

Parsnip juice is a traditional remedy for beautifying the skin, hair, and nails.

Wheatgrass Juice: The Number-One Antiaging Hero

Wheatgrass juice proponents claim that it increases hemoglobin production, rebuilds the bloodstream, purifies the blood, improves the body's ability to heal wounds, creates an unfavorable environment for *Candida albicans* growth, cleanses drug deposits from the body, and neutralizes toxins and carcinogens in the body. It is also said to help purify the liver, lower blood pressure, and improve blood sugar metabolism.

Wheatgrass is grown, first by soaking wheat berries overnight, then planting them, usually in a tray with about two inches of soil, and letting them grow until the shoots are about seven inches high. The wheatgrass is then cut, rinsed, and forced through a special juice extractor to glean the rich, green juice from the tender shoots. The chlorophyll-rich cocktail is drunk immediately after juicing, one or two ounces at a time, two times a day, for the most benefit.

Many health food stores, juice bars, and natural foods restaurants offer wheatgrass juice by the one- or two-ounce shot. Or you can purchase flats of wheatgrass at many whole foods markets or grow it at home and juice your own. A high-quality manual wheatgrass juicer can be purchased for less than $200; a good electric juicer can cost as much as $600. Whichever route you may go, the health and antiaging benefits of wheatgrass juice are worth the money and the time it takes to acquire.

It is best always to drink wheatgrass juice immediately after it is made to get the most benefit. Some people like its taste; most do not. If you don't like it, it is encouraging to know that you only have to consume it in small doses and can swig it down quickly. Some people chase it with a little lemon water or chew a few fresh herb leaves, although the most benefit is derived in drinking it on an empty stomach with nothing consumed before or afterward for at least thirty minutes.

Ann's Story

The late Ann Wigmore, known as the pioneer of wheatgrass juicing, the raw foods movement, and sprouting, and the author of *The Wheatgrass Book,* was a fabulous advertisement for the antiaging effects of cleansing the body and feeding it a high-nutrient, enzyme-rich diet that included lots of wheatgrass juice. At age fifty, she was ill, had an injury that was not healing, with gangrene setting in that threatened amputation, was chronically fatigued, gray-haired, and looked older than her years. She started experimenting with raw foods and changed her lifestyle. Within a short time her fatigue, illnesses, and even the gangrene vanished. Her gray hair returned to its original dark color and her skin tightened as though she'd had a face-lift. Her energy increased and her health returned.

Ann Wigmore was the forerunner of a growing number of individuals who have experienced firsthand a reversal of signs of aging by incorporating many of the foods and juices Ann touted. Scores of nutrition-oriented clinics of Europe and a number of health institutes in the United States support Ann's findings that a diet focused on nutrient-dense foods such as raw vegetables, sprouts, and vegetable juices promote healing of many degenerative diseases associated with aging. Thousands of people in America have experienced the healing, restorative power of this kind of diet, promoted at a number of health institutes from coast to coast.

Adding wheatgrass juice and other high-antioxidant juices, raw foods, and sprouts into your diet is easy and the rewards are enormous. With these live foods, you're on your way to a healthier, younger looking you. (See Resources, p. 254, for centers that offer live foods programs.)

GRAINS

To avoid free radical damage to cells, blood sugar imbalance, and inflammation caused by refined flour products, choose only whole grains such as oatmeal (not instant), amaranth, millet, brown and wild rice (a grass), and quinoa as the healthiest grains for cooking, baking, and breakfast cereal. Avoid all white rice. Eliminate wheat as much as possible; it's been widely overused in this country and many people are sensitive or allergic as a result. Look for whole organic grains at your health food store. When it comes to flour, it's best to grind your own whenever possible. Flour that sits on shelves in bags is prone to molds, which cause inflammation.

Wrinkle Cleanse Whole Grains and Cereal Grass

All whole grains are beneficial, but especially include:

Amaranth	Rye
Barley	Quinoa
Millet	Spelt
Oatmeal (not instant)	Wild rice (cereal grass)
Rice (brown rice of all types)	

NUTS AND SEEDS

Most nuts and seeds contain 15 to 25 percent protein combined with fat (about 50 to 60 percent) and carbohydrate (25 to 35 percent). They are a good source of some of the B vitamins and a variety of minerals. Nuts and seeds are best eaten in small portions, if you're watching your weight, because they are high in calories. They make good snacks "on the run" since they are easy to carry and provide quality blood sugar–stabilizing nutrients.

The healthiest nuts and seeds are grown organically and can be found at most health food stores. It's best to buy raw nuts whenever possible and keep them refrigerated. Or try one of my favorites—tamari almonds; they're really delicious and available at many whole foods markets. Commercial nuts often have been heated in refined oils that are not part of the Wrinkle Cleanse Diet, so it's best to avoid them. And dry roasted nuts aren't much better; they usually are coated with a variety of additives.

You may want to consider soaking seeds and nuts in water overnight (six to eight hours for seeds; ten to twelve hours for nuts). Soaking promotes *germination* (the beginning process of growth). During germination the seed or nut springs to life, increasing its nutritional potential; enzyme inhibitors are removed and predigestion occurs, increasing digestability. In the predigestion phase, starches are converted into simple sugars, proteins are broken down into amino acids, and fats are converted into more usable fatty acids.

For soaking, all you need is a jar and filtered or distilled water. When the soaking time is up, drain the water and rinse the nuts or seeds well. If you want them crunchy, place the seeds or nuts in a dehydrator with a temperature that is not over 118°F (to preserve the enzymes) and dehydrate until crunchy. Nuts and seeds prepared this way are very delicious, but best of all, they are the healthiest. Dehydrated in this manner, they are considered a raw food.

Wrinkle Cleanse Nuts and Seeds*

Almonds	Pecans
Brazil nuts	Pine nuts
Cashews	Pistachios
Hazelnuts	Pumpkin seeds
Macadamia nuts	Sesame seeds
Peanuts (actually not a nut— a legume)	Sunflower seeds
	Walnuts

*Other healthy choices include the butters made from these nuts like almond or macadamia nut butter and the pastes made from seeds such as tahini made from sesame seeds.

FRUIT

Fruit is cleansing and contains an abundance of antioxidants and other important vitamins, minerals, enzymes, and phytochemicals. It's important to limit its consumption, however, because of its natural sugars. It's best to eat only small amounts of fruit at one time and average two servings a day, avoiding the high-sugar fruit (see p. 50). Fruit juice should be limited or avoided because of its high sugar content, with the exception of lemon or lime, low-sugar apple such as pippin or Granny Smith, and berries. You can add the juice of half of a low-sugar apple such as Granny Smith or pippin or lemon to vegetable juice for flavor enhancement.

Berries such as blueberries, blackberries, and raspberries are low in sugar, making them an excellent choice. And they have not been subjected to the hybridization process like many other fruits, which has allowed them to maintain their small size and low sugar content. They are the richest fruit in many phytochemicals like flavonoids and anthocyanidins. Blueberries in particular have been shown in research to reverse certain aging characteristics. One study showed that old rats fed the equivalent of one cup of blueberries a day were smarter and more coordinated than other old rats. Also, rats fed spinach and strawberries learned better than rats on a standard rodent diet. The most protective compounds in berries, which make strawberries red and blueberries blue, are known as anthocyanins. It is believed that these compounds may reduce inflammation, which is also very important in the fight against aging.

Though not thought of as fruit, other good fruit choices include avocado and tomato. Avocado is an excellent source of essential fatty acids, glutathione (a powerful antioxidant), and amino acids. It contains more potassium than bananas (which are not recommended because of their high sugar content) making them an excellent choice for the heart. And tomatoes are one of the richest sources of vitamin C and lycopene. Lycopene is a carotenoid that exhibits the most powerful singlet-oxygen (free radical) subduing abilities.

It is best to avoid watermelon, bananas, grapes, pineapple, oranges, and all dried fruit as much as possible since they are among the highest sugar-containing fruits.

Wrinkle Cleanse Fruit

LOW-SUGAR FRUIT

Avocado	Cranberries
Apple (pippin or Granny Smith is best)	Grapefruit
	Lemon
Berries: blueberries, blackberries, raspberries, strawberries	Lime
	Tomato

MODERATELY SWEET FRUIT (should be consumed in smaller amounts)

Apples: sweeter apples such as
    Red and Golden Delicious and
    applesauce
Apricot
Cantaloupe
Crenshaw
Cherries
Figs (fresh)
Guava
Honeydew
Kiwi
Kumquat
Loquat
Lychees

Mango
Melons
Nectarine
Orange
Papaya
Passion fruit
Peach
Pear
Persimmon
Plum
Pomegranate
Rhubarb
Tangerine

HIGH-SUGAR FRUIT

Bananas
Dried fruit
Grapes
Pineapple
Watermelon

FATS AND OILS

In recent decades, fat has been the bad guy, but thanks to the low-carb diet gurus, fat has taken its rightful place in society again. Fat gives rich flavor to food. It adds satiety to a meal—a feeling of having had enough to eat. And now we're learning that it isn't the heart disease culprit we once thought. Often, people who avoid all fat just don't feel like they've had enough to eat, even when the volume of food consumed has been more than enough. Fat-free and low-fat foods are one of the reasons some people overeat carbohydrates, which really packs on the pounds and sets us up for insulin resistance and inflammation.

A diet of whole foods will be a high-fat diet. Grains that contain all of their components, which we call *whole grains,* will be rich in oils. It is virtually impossible to eliminate fats from our food unless we refine them. Fats are an essential part of life; without them, we could not survive. Four vitamins—A, D, E, and K—are fat-soluble vitamins, meaning they are soluble in fat and fat transports them in our body. When fat is removed from a food, many of the fat-soluble vitamins and other healthful components are also removed and the carrier of fat-soluble vitamins is unavailable.

What's a healthful fat, and what is not, is part of the great debate on fat these days. There's a lot of very confusing information circulating and often it's tough to make sense of the whole thing. One point few health professionals disagree on, however, is the necessity of eating ample amounts of healthy fats known as the essential fatty acids. Unsaturated omega-3 and omega-6 fatty acids are called essential because the body cannot manufacture them; we must get them from our diet. And though we need only small amounts, without them our health suffers.

Good fats like the omega-3 fatty acids are vital to the health of our skin, hair, nails, heart, and brain. Good fats are very important in prevention of wrinkles, dry skin, and skin problems such as eczema. Without good fats, our hair would look like straw, our nails would peel, and our skin would become dry, scaly, and wrinkled. Essential fats prevent oxidation of keratin (a tough protein substance in hair and nails). Eating a low-fat or no-fat diet will, over time, produce visible signs of aging. But that's not all—a diet deficient in good fats will starve our heart and joints and make us more susceptible to cancer. The body was designed for fat—healthy fats.

The essential fatty acids (EFAs) must be obtained from foods such as fatty coldwater fish, cod liver oil, and flaxseeds; the body cannot make them. The omega-3 fatty acids are known to stop inflammation within the body and are exceptionally good at halting pro-inflammatory chemicals made inside the body from unhealthy fats, which means they help curb inflammation that contributes to microscarring and thus to wrinkles and lines.

The Beauty Oils Glossary

A number of fats and oils can make a huge improvement in how you look—from lackluster to shiny hair; dry, dull skin to glowing; brittle to strong nails; and from pudgy to trim body. The Beauty Oils Glossary can help you incorporate into your diet the oils that can work wonders from the inside out. And remember, it's far better to consume these oils than simply to rub them on your skin. A small amount is absorbed externally, but when ingested, these oils can make a big difference in how you look from the inside out.

Coconut Oil

Coconut oil is one of the most slimming oils you can eat. It is comprised predominantly of short- and medium-chain triglycerides (molecules of fatty acids) that the body likes to burn; they act a lot like kindling in a fire rather than a big, damp log. The body does not readily deposit these fatty acids in adipose tissue (fat cells), but rather sends them directly to the liver, where they're used for fuel. They are a bit like using premium fuel in your car, rather than a cheap grade gasoline. Also, tropical oils such as coconut and palm oils have about one and a half fewer calories per gram of fat compared with other oils such as soy, corn, or safflower oils. Coconut oil also helps the skin look silky smooth and the hair shiny. For extra glow, rub coconut oil on your skin and hair before you shampoo.

EVENING PRIMROSE OIL

Rich in omega-6 fatty acids, with significant levels of gamma-linolenic acid (GLA, a derivative of linoleic acid), evening primrose oil is known as an essential fatty acid (EFA). It is called *essential* because the body cannot produce it. Evening primrose oil is helpful for brittle nails and dry eyes. It helps lower triglycerides and LDL cholesterol and improves a cell's sensitivity to insulin. When combined with zinc, it is also helpful in treating acne. And it has another bonus: It has been shown in scientific studies to improve PMS symptoms. You can find it at most health food stores.

FISH OIL

Some of the best fats for our skin and hair are the oils found in fish. Fish oils are rich in essential fatty acids (EFAs) and especially EPA (eicosapentaenoic acid) and DHA (docosahexaenoic acid). Without EFAs, our hair looks dry and breaks easily, and may even fall out. Nails become dry and brittle. And when we don't eat enough of these fats, our skin appears dull, feels dry or scaly, and doesn't glow with health; even wounds may not heal easily. Omega-3 fatty acids can be found in abundance in fatty coldwater fish such as salmon, mackerel, tuna, sardines, shad, and trout and in fish oils such as cod liver oil, which is also a very good source of vitamin A—a "beautiful skin" vitamin. (You can buy flavored cod liver oil, which helps improve the taste, at health food stores.) EFAs are also prevalent in flaxseeds and flax oil.

FLAXSEEDS AND FLAXSEED OIL

Flaxseeds and oil are rich in EFAs, which make the skin feel and look velvety and glowing. Skin nourished well from within with EFAs is smoother, looks softer, and is more radiant. It also ages more slowly and remains wrinkle-free longer. Look for unrefined, cold-pressed flaxseed oil and flaxseeds at health food stores. This oil is quite perishable, and needs to be refrigerated at all times; it should be kept no longer than three months.

Hemp Seeds and Hemp Oil

Hemp seeds and oil contain the essential fatty acids (EFAs) omega-6 and omega-3 in ideal ratios of three to one. They are also very good for the skin, and do many of the good things flaxseeds and oil do in the body.

Olive Oil

Mediterranean people are known for their beautiful, glowing skin and their diet is rich in extra-virgin olive oil. Olive oil contains oleic acid, a member of the omega-9 fatty acids. A very stable monounsaturate, olive oil is associated with a wide range of health and beauty benefits. Regularly using olive oil can mean the difference between skin that looks like leather and skin that is soft and glowing. The best olive oil is extra virgin, which comes from the first pressing of olives. (Avocado and nuts such as almond and macadamia are also good sources of oleic acid.)

We need the omega-3 fatty acids because they reduce the production of inflammatory agents within our bodies, which contribute to aging. Eicosanoid acid, the most potent inflammation-causing compound, is produced in the body from the linoleic acid that comes from margarine, shortening, and refined vegetable oils. Omega-3 fatty acids actually stop production of eiconsanoid acid. (Reducing our consumption of foods, such as most vegetable oils, that are high in linoleic acid is the best line of defense.)

Not only is getting enough omega-3s important; the ratio of omega-3 to omega-6 fatty acid consumption is also essential. Consumption of omega-3s has decreased drastically in the last century, while omega-6s have more than doubled in our food supply. Polyunsaturated fatty acids (PUFAs), which are rich in omega-6s, are abundant in the typical American diet. Researchers tell us these fatty acids should be limited to about 5 percent of the diet, and the ratio of omega-6 to omega-3 consumption should be from two-to-one to three-to-one. Many people get far too many omega-6s, which, when contributing to an imbalanced ratio with omega-3s, contributes to aging and degenerative disease. And this in turn has an impact on the makeup of the cells of our body, which leads to poor cellular construction.

Alpha-linolenic acid (not to be confused with linoleic acid) is an important omega-3 and is found in dark green leafy vegetables; flaxseeds and oil; hemp seeds and oil; and coldwater fish such as salmon, herring, mackerel, sardines, shad, and trout, and fish oil. Wild caught salmon is one of the richest sources of EPA (eicosapentaenoic acid) and DHA (docosahexaenoic acid), two of the most beneficial of the alpha-linolenic acids. These fats remind the body to "turn off" inflammatory reactions when they are no longer needed. Note, however, that farm-raised salmon are not a good source of omega-3s since their diet is deficient in marine foods that produce the omega-3s in the fish.

Another important anti-inflammatory fatty acid is known as GLA (gamma-linolenic acid) and is found in certain seeds—borage, black current, and evening primrose. (Most supplemental forms of GLA are derived from these seeds.) Consuming vegetable oils such as corn, safflower, sunflower, or soy can interfere with the conversion of linoleic acid to GLA. Supplemental GLA boosts the production of DGLA, the precursor of prostaglandin E1, which suppresses inflammation. These fats also help to lower cortisol and norepinephrine, hormones released during times of stress, which contribute to inflammation and weight gain.

THE BEST OILS AND FATS FOR FOOD PREPARATION

The polyunsaturated fats have been hailed as healthy for decades, but now we're learning that they aren't the healthiest after all. These vegetable oils are unstable and can easily turn to rancid fat (a process called oxidation), which generates free radicals. When free radicals attack the connective tissue that holds our skin together and gives it suppleness and elasticity, the fibers break down and our skin wrinkles and sags.

Two oils—olive and coconut oils—are far more resistant to this happening and are recommended for the Wrinkle Cleanse Diet food preparation. Oleic acid is the basic building block of omega-9 fatty acids and is found in olive oil, macadamia nuts and oil, and avocados. Though the body can make omega-9 fatty acids from other fats, these foods supply a direct source of this very beneficial fatty acid. Omega-9s are excellent fats for the skin and have demonstrated anti-inflammatory properties. Also, many of the benefits of the heart healthy diet of the Mediterranean people can be attributed to olive oil. Olives from Spain are said to have the highest content of *polyphenolic flavonoids* (phytochemicals with antioxidant activity) that slow the aging process.

Olive oil is called *virgin* if it is extracted by means of pressure from millstones and is not treated with heat or chemicals. Batches of olives are pressed more than once to produce numerous batches of oil. The first pressing of the olives produces *extra-virgin* oil, which is the most flavorful and has the least acidity and the highest amount of fatty acids and polyphenols (antioxidants).

Extra-virgin olive oil made from olives organically grown in the Mediterranean is the healthiest choice. Olive oil is best for salad dressings and recipes that don't require cooking. Olive oil can be used for sautéing on low heat, and is sometimes most desirable for flavor in certain cooked recipes, but is best used for cold food preparation.

Coconut oil is one of the most stable oils for cooking. Coconut oil has no double carbon bonds—the weak links that are vulnerable to free radical attack and easily broken—making it much more stable under a variety of conditions such as heat, light, moisture, and oxygen without undergoing oxidation (rancidity). Typically, it can sit on shelves in the sweltering temperatures of the tropics for up to two years without turning rancid.

People who regularly use coconut oil often report that their skin becomes softer and more glowing. Just recently my neighbor, who started cooking with coconut oil several weeks before, asked me if the oil could be the reason his rough elbows were suddenly becoming smooth. Coconut oil was the only explanation I had because it was the only change he'd made in his diet. One only needs to look at the skin of many Polynesian and Asian women who eat a traditional diet rich in coconut oil to find proof that it, along with their traditional whole foods, has a profound smoothing and nourishing effect on their skin.

Coconut oil has received considerable bad press in recent years due to a media campaign designed to discredit tropical oils. That premise is not founded in truth but on studies performed decades ago and a lot of supposition since. (If you want to read more about this, see my website www.gococonuts.com.)

Coconut oil is believed to enhance thyroid function. This in turn stimulates the conversion of low-density lipoprotein cholesterol into the antiaging hormones pregneonolone, progesterone, and dehydroepiandrosterone (DHEA). These valuable hormones not only aid in antiaging and weight management, but also in preventing heart disease, senility, and other degenerative diseases. It is believed that coconut helps correct sluggish thyroid function that causes weight gain, hair loss, insomnia, and low energy by supporting the conversion of T4 to T3 (thyroid hormones).

Just as with olive oil, be choosy when it comes to coconut oil. Many commercial grade coconut oils are made from copra, the unrefined dried kernel (meat) of the coconut. Though producers may start with organic coconuts and even label their coconut oil organic, they subject the oil from copra to heat and a chemical refining process that results in bleached and deodorized oil. Standard copra-based oils often have a sour taste and smell and can really turn you off to using coconut oil.

But, if you use virgin coconut oil made the "old-fashioned way," you will immediately notice the difference in taste, smell (delicate fragrance), color (whiter), and texture compared with other coconut oils. It may cost more, but it's well worth it.

Macadamia nut oil is also a good choice for food preparation, but is difficult to find. Sesame oil and peanut oil can be used in small quantities. Butter is the only other fat that I recommend for cooking, but it should be used sparingly. Raw, cultured butter from dairy cows that have been raised free-range and grass fed is your healthiest choice; it is rich in vitamin A, selenium, and conjugated linoleic acid (CLA).

Wrinkle Cleanse Fats and Oils*

Butter (organic; use
   sparingly)
Coconut oil (virgin is best)
Macadamia nut oil (cold
   pressed)
Olive oil (cold pressed,
   extra virgin is best)

Peanut oil (cold pressed,
   small quantities)
Sesame oil (cold pressed,
   small quantities)

*Organic for all oils is healthiest.

PROTEIN

After water, protein is the most plentiful substance in the body. It is an integral part of every living cell—the building blocks of the animal kingdom. Complete proteins are combinations of twenty-two amino acids, of which eleven are considered essential, meaning we must get them from our food. Amino acids are necessary for building and repair. Enzymes are specialized proteins, as are antibodies. When we don't eat enough protein for cellular repair, we won't have healthy-looking, wrinkle-free, taut skin and strong, healthy hair and nails.

Protein is necessary for repairing cells damaged by free radical attack. A lack of protein prevents cellular repair and accelerates the aging process. The sulfur-containing amino acids—methionine, cysteine, and cystine—are particularly important to the skin. Sulfur plays an important role in collagen integrity and healthy skin, hair, and nails. For example, methionine helps prevent brittle hair that breaks easily. Cysteine is formed from methionine in the presence of vitamin B_6; it protects collagen from damage and makes the skin more flexible. Cystine, which aids in the formation of skin and is important in detoxification, is easily converted from cysteine.

Protein also stimulates the production of glucagon, a substance that stimulates the breakdown of glycogen and the release of glucose by the liver. When synchronized, insulin and glucagon create a stable hormonal system, which is significant in preventing premature aging.

Digestion of protein is crucial to its utilization. Stomach acid (hydrochloric acid) starts declining around age forty. Without enough strong acids in the stomach to digest protein, pancreatic enzymes can't effectively handle the increased work that is necessary. That means some undigested protein will make its way through the system into the intestines. There in the warm moist folds bacteria "lie in wait" for the incompletely digested morsels. When the two meet bacterial digestion takes place, a process known as putrefaction, and toxins are produced, many of which are absorbed into the bloodstream. These toxins can cause our skin tone to deteriorate, our nails to grow weak, and our hair to break. If you are over forty, I recommend that you take a supplement called

Protein Powder

Protein powder can be a good supplement in the diet, if it's a healthy choice. Added to a breakfast smoothie, for example, or for a mid-morning or afternoon pick-me-up healthy shake, protein powder can give the body a boost in energy. And this can make a difference in how we look and feel. If we don't get enough protein, our skin suffers like the rest of our body. There are days when eating on the run may not provide the protein we need. Hence, protein powder to the rescue!

The type of protein powder we choose is very important. I recommend rice or whey protein powder (dairy or goat), but not soy protein powder due to a growing concern that too much soy in the diet can negatively affect thyroid health. (Soy is a goitrogen, meaning that it blocks iodine absorption.) One particular protein powder, Ultra InflamX, a rice protein–based powder, is known as a medical food. It is helpful to reduce inflammation throughout the body and it contains some excellent anti-inflammatory ingredients such as turmeric and ginger root.

betaine HCl to assist in protein digestion and counteract these effects on your skin, nails, and hair.

Women who aren't exceptionally active need about 60 grams of protein each day; men typically need 80 to 90 grams. It's important to choose protein wisely. I recommend leaner cuts of meat or poultry since animals tend to store toxins more in fat cells than muscle. The best protein choices are wild-caught fish and naturally raised, organically fed poultry. In order to get valuable iron, you may benefit from a little free-range red meat occasionally (once or twice a month, but no more than once a week). Free-range animals that have been grass fed and raised without antibiotics and hormones provide meat that is much higher in the very beneficial conjugated linoleic acid (CLA). Cage-free eggs are also an excellent source of protein, especially the sulfur-rich amino acids. Dairy products should be limited as much as possible.

A Note to Vegetarians

Complete proteins are found only in animal products; incomplete proteins are in plant foods. Vegetarians can get a balance of proteins from consuming a wide variety of plant foods such as legumes (beans, lentils, split peas), whole grains, dark greens, sprouts, and sea vegetables. But it's much harder to get all the amino acids one needs from just plant foods. Vegetarians have to work hard at getting the right balance and many don't succeed. A deficiency of protein can show up in sagging, wrinkled skin; sugar cravings; and depressed immunity resulting in more infections.

Fish is an excellent source of protein and good fats. Fatty, coldwater fish is especially loaded with healthy fats, namely the omega-3 fatty acids and especially EPA (eicosapentaenoic acid) and DHA (docosahexaenoic acid). Choose smaller, coldwater fish such as salmon, sardines, mackerel, shad, and trout as they are richer in omega-3s and have less mercury then larger fish such as swordfish, bass, and tuna. Avoid farm-raised salmon (and other farm-raised fish and seafood) because of the added dyes applied to mask their rather gray flesh (salmon) and the antibiotics given them to help them fight infection due to overcrowding and unsanitary "water pen" conditions.

Wild-caught salmon is not only one of nature's best sources of omega-3 fatty acids, it's also rich in DMAE, an antioxidant known to cause muscles to contract and tighten. Improving muscle contractions helps your facial muscles, giving you fewer bags and sags and more contours! You may want to take a DMAE nutritional supplement for an extra boost of antisagging action. You'll also get another bonus with DMAE—it is good for the brain; it can help you think more clearly. No wonder they call fish and seafood "brain food"!

Whenever possible, choose antibiotic-free and organically raised poultry. The growth hormones injected into factory farm-raised animals can cause them to gain weight quickly, which is good for getting them to market early. But these hormone and antibiotic residues in the animal's flesh are not healthful; there's indication that they adversely affect the health of the humans that eat them.

Eggs are an excellent protein source. They contain the essential amino acids including the sulfur-rich amino acids that are so good for the skin. They are also a rich source of essential fatty acids (EFAs). (See The Beauty Oils Glossary, p. 53, for more information on EFAs.) They also contain considerably more lecithin (a fat emulsifier) than cholesterol; phosphatidylcholine (present in lecithin) is used nutritionally to treat high cholesterol. (That fact should dispel the fear about eggs and cholesterol.) They are also rich in sulfur (a chemical involved in hair and nails development), choline (a brain nutrient, particularly a memory enhancer), and glutathione (a powerful antioxidant). Choose eggs from chickens raised cage-free and fed an organic diet.

Choose free-range, grass-fed beef whenever possible in order to get appreciable amounts of CLA (conjugated linoleic acid). This is a fatty acid that we must get from our food because the body cannot produce it. CLA has been shown to promote weight loss by normalizing body fat deposition and to prevent cancer. Limit red meat to no more than one serving per week.

Natural foods markets such as Whole Foods and Wild Oats and many independent health food stores and local farmers markets offer grass-fed, naturally raised, organically fed, and hormone-free beef, lamb, buffalo, poultry products, and eggs from cage-free, organically fed chickens.

When it comes to animal fat, it is recommend that you keep it to a minimum. Animals are higher on the food chain and tend to store toxins in fat cells more than muscle. Though choosing organically raised animal products is far superior to factory farm–raised animals that are grown in crowded, unhealthy conditions and given antibiotics and hormones, toxins will still be stored in the fat, because it is almost impossible to avoid them these days.

Though protein is important, none of us need to eat animal protein every day. Animal protein is heavy and considered a building food. Many Americans eat too much, which leads to overacidity in the body and is hard on the kidneys. To counteract these effects, I recommended that with each change of season, you take a number of cleansing days where you avoid all animal products. I also recommend one vegetarian day a week, or a vegetable juice fast day (one day a week), or the two-day raw food rejuvenator—raw plant–based days. These are all days that will give your system a rest from the intense work of digesting animal proteins. In general, vegetarian days will give your system an abundance of antioxidants and a chance to gently flush away some toxins. As a result, you should experience improved digestion and more vibrant, younger-looking skin.

Wrinkle Cleanse Lean Animal Proteins

Fish of all types (wild-caught is best)
Poultry (choose cage-free, antibiotic- and hormone-free, organically fed)
    Chicken: skinless breast and thighs are best
    Cornish game hens
    Turkey: skinless is best
    Turkey bacon; turkey ham

DAIRY

Dairy products are a good source of protein, riboflavin, vitamin D, and calcium. It is debated that the calcium in dairy may not be as absorbable as that in dark leafy greens, especially kale, parsley, and watercress; nuts such as almonds, Brazil nuts, and walnuts; and sunflower and sesame seeds and tahini (sesame paste). The healthiest dairy choices are products that come from free-range, organically fed cows. If you can't find organic products, at least make sure the ones you choose are not from cows given BGH (bovine growth hormone). (This is not easy because manufacturers are not required to list this hormone.) Plain organic yogurt is the best dairy choice since it contains good bacteria for the intestinal tract. (If you have to take a round of antibiotics, always follow with plain organic yogurt, kefir, or probiotics; all contain good bacteria to replace the beneficial intestinal bacteria destroyed by the antibiotics.)

Goat cheese and other goat milk products may be better tolerated than dairy cow products. When it comes to dairy cheese, feta, Parmesan, and Romano are among the best choices; use in small amounts for added flavor in salads, omelets, and frittatas. It is best to limit dairy products for your Wrinkle Cleanse lifestyle.

Wrinkle Cleanse Dairy Foods

Feta	Ricotta cheese
Goat cheese	Romano
Kefir	Parmesan
Mozzarella	Plain organic yogurt

WATER

Water is as important to our bodies as oil is to our cars. In fact, it's critical to the functioning of every cell and organ in the body. It is significant for the fluid content of the blood and acts as a medium to carry electrical charges through the body like a telephone wire carries signals. It's important for hormone and neurotransmitter conduction, and it transports nutrients to cells. Water is also vital to cleansing every organ and system in our body, enabling it to flush out toxins.

Without water we would die. The body is 70 percent to 75 percent water, and the brain is made up of about 50 percent water. It is estimated that many Americans over forty are running at a water deficit, with closer to 60 percent water in their body. F. Batmanghelidj, MD, author of *Your Body's Many Cries for Water,* says, "chronic cellular dehydration painfully and prematurely kills. Its initial outward manifestations have, until now, been labeled diseases of unknown origin."

Stephen Cherniske, MS, nutrition consultant, health educator, and researcher, says, "Americans consume more coffee and soft drinks [both dehydrating] than water. If you do this you might as well paste a sign on your forehead, *Aging as fast as I can.*"

To age as slowly as possible, hydrate your skin so it looks dewy and soft by drinking plenty of water. It is also important to limit coffee and alcohol (both dehydrating), avoid soft drinks completely, and drink a minimum of eight to ten glasses of water each and every day. If you do on occasion drink coffee or an alcoholic beverage, follow with a glass of water for every cup of coffee or alcoholic drink you consume. And start carrying water bottles everywhere you go so you're always able to drink to a younger you.

A Word About Dehydration

Some people avoid drinking water for fear of water retention. But it isn't drinking water that causes this phenomenon; it is often the lack of it. When we're dehydrated, which many people are, the body will retain water. If you wait until you are thirsty to drink water, you are already dehydrated. Fitness instructors constantly remind us of this fact and also that our metabolism drops slightly when we are dehydrated. If you ever had questions about the benefits of drinking water, just drop a prune in a glass of water and watch what happens. Leave it there for a few hours and—I bet you already know what happens—it starts looking more like a plum again. Water has a similar effect on your body and your face.

BEVERAGES

The best beverages for wrinkle cleansing aren't the ones you see advertised often. Herbal tea, green tea, sparkling mineral water, vegetable juices, and, of course pure water are important components of the Wrinkle Cleanse Diet. These beverages hydrate the body and contribute to better health.

Green tea and herbal tea are far better choices than coffee. Green tea is especially healthful. Not only is it rich in the antioxidant catechin polyphenol, which protects us against inflammation, cancer, and other ailments, it is also a known *thermogenic*. Thermogenesis is the production of heat, which revs up the metabolism and promotes weight loss. And a cup of green tea has about a third of the caffeine found in a cup of coffee.

If you are caffeine sensitive or have low adrenal or thyroid function or are hypoglycemic, it is best to avoid caffeinated green tea as well as all other caffeine-containing products such as coffee, black tea, soda pop, and chocolate, which aren't part of the Wrinkle Cleanse Diet, but are especially detrimental for people with those conditions. When choosing green and herbal tea, look for the healthiest tea, which is organically grown. Also, unbleached tea bags are better choices over bleached.

Sparkling mineral water (such as S. Pellegrino and Apollinaris) that is naturally carbonated, rather than commercially gassed, is the best choice and will provide some minerals. Freshly made vegetable juices from organic produce are always healthier than bottled or canned. When choosing canned or bottled juice, such as tomato or V-8, choose low-sodium and organic, if available.

Wrinkle Cleanse Beverages

Green tea (organic, unbleached tea bags are best); omit if you have
   thyroid or adrenal challenges or are hypoglycemic
Herbal tea (organic, unbleached tea bags are best); serve hot and iced
Sparkling mineral water (naturally carbonated) with lemon or lime or
   unsweetened cranberry or black cherry juice concentrate for flavor
Freshly made vegetable juices, organic is best

SWEETENERS

Since most sugars contribute to the aging process, it is best to choose those that don't significantly affect blood sugar levels. (See Chapter 3, p. 76, for more information.) There are three low-carb healthy sweeteners that I recommend: stevia, birch sugar (xylitol), and Lo Han Guo.

Stevia is extracted from an herbal leaf of a plant that comes from

South America. It is about two to three hundred times sweeter than sugar, so you need only a small amount in comparison to sugar. It has virtually no calories and there is no evidence that it is harmful to the body in any way. The FDA does not allow it to be marketed as a sweetener, but rather it is labeled as a nutritional supplement. Stevia comes in powdered or liquid form and also in packets; it can be found at most health food stores.

Birch sugar (xylitol) is a sugar alcohol. The healthiest xylitol is derived from birch bark. It has fewer calories than sugar with about the same sweetness. It has not been shown to promote tooth decay, and it is metabolized slowly, which helps prevent the sugar highs and lows often experienced with other sweeteners. When buying birch sugar, be aware that not all brands are made from birch trees; much of what we see in stores today is made from pulp waste from the paper industry and should be avoided. Read labels to determine the source. You can also look for one reliable source called the Ultimate Sweetener. (See Resources, p. 250.)

Lo Han Guo comes from the Chinese plant Lo Han Guo, *Siraitia grosvenorii,* a perennial vine in the cucumber-melon family that grows in China. Lo Han fruits contain triterpene glycoside sweeteners known as mogrosides. When processed into a fine powder, this natural sweetener is soluble in water. Like stevia, it is about three hundred times sweeter than sugar, so very little is needed to sweeten foods and beverages. It is also very low in calories.

Wrinkle Cleanse Sweeteners

Birch sugar (xylitol)
Lo Han Guo
Stevia

CELTIC SEA SALT

Whole sea salt, known as Celtic salt or gray salt, has a mineral profile that is similar to our blood. In Chinese medicine, whole sea salt is known for its detoxifying properties and is thought to have a grounding effect that leads to clarity of mind, when used in moderation. A pinch of Celtic salt in warm water has been said to help people get to sleep at night—a big boon for looking rested and younger. Celtic salt can be found at most health food stores.

Substances That Accelerate Aging

I t's exciting to learn about what we can add to our diet and lifestyle to look younger and reverse signs of aging, and though it is always fun to find out about the foods and nutrients we can include, it is equally important to know what we need to omit to prevent premature aging. The foods and substances reviewed in this chapter are the ones known to contribute to the aging process.

Certain substances will cause the body to age faster and make it more susceptible to skin damage, because they deplete it of nutrients, cause oxidation in cells, and contribute to inflammation. Many such substances contribute to the body's toxic burden and stress the liver and other organs of elimination. These substances include caffeine, alcohol, tobacco, artificial flavorings and colorings, preservatives, nitrates, nitrites, recreational drugs, many prescription drugs, refined salt, sugar, sugar substitutes, damaged fats, refined flour products, high-carb foods, pesticides, and environmental toxins.

If we don't minimize these substances, or better yet eliminate them, from our diet and lifestyle (and cleanse them from our body periodically), they will eventually contribute to disease. Therefore, it's as important for our faces as it is for our health that we look at the substances that accelerate aging.

The Simple Carbohydrates

Carbohydrates are macronutrients known as sugars, starches, and fiber. They are composed of carbon, hydrogen, and oxygen and are formed when carbon dioxide and water combine in the presence of sunlight and chlorophyll (green or purple pigment in plants). The chemical bonds of the carbohydrate lock in the energy of the sun. This energy is released when we burn carbs for fuel.

Carbs come arranged in three sizes—monosaccharides, disaccharides, or polysaccharides. Sugars with a single sugar ring, such as glucose, fructose, and galactose are known as monosaccharides and sugars made from pairs of single rings, such as sucrose, lactose, and maltose are known as disaccharides (the simple carbohydrates). Sugar, fruit juice, and white bread are examples of simple carbs. Large molecules known as starches, glycogen (found in animal meats to a limited extent), and fiber are long chains of single-ring sugars linked together. They are known as polysaccharides or the complex carbohydrates. Vegetables, beans, and whole grains are some of the most healthful, fiber-rich examples of complex carbohydrates.

REFINED CARBOHYDRATES AND HIGH-CARB FOODS

Though we need carbohydrates in our diet for energy, we don't need refined carbs and high-carb foods. These carbs contribute to aging and disease. Refined carbohydrates are foods that have had some of their most important elements removed in processing. For example, grains processed into fluffy white flour have had the bran, germ, and chaff removed, along with many minerals and vitamins, and they are bleached to make them white. Refined flour products easily convert to sugar in the body, which contributes to blood sugar imbalances that can lead to insulin resistance and inflammation. White sugar that has been refined from sugarcane or beets has had minerals and fiber stripped away; it is also made white by bleaching. (Bleach residues can be toxic.)

Some of the high-carbohydrate foods that contribute to insulin spikes can catch us off guard—they don't taste sweet, and we may think we're actually eating something healthful. Take a rice cake, for example. It has no fat and not a lot of calories, but look out when it comes to carbs— about twelve carbs in each flavored rice cake; about eight carb grams in the plain ones. Many people have felt good about eating several rice cakes for a snack in place of something that contains fat, but they are not a good-carb choice. They are made of puffed rice, which is high on the glycemic index (an index that shows the rate at which carbohydrates break down to glucose in the bloodstream and turn to sugar). Other high-carb foods that are high on the glycemic index include potatoes, white rice, corn, refined grain products, sugar, and sweets.

When grains are refined, they are stripped of precious minerals such as zinc, chromium, and manganese, which help control blood sugar levels, and the fiber that helps stabilize blood sugar and promote good elimination. Also, grains that have been ground into fine flour and sit on a shelf in bags are prone to molds—a potent source of free radicals that contribute to inflammation and oxidation (damaged cells). And to make matters worse, overeating a particular food like refined wheat can cause a sensitivity or allergy to that food, which contributes to inflammation.

Most of us have grown up overeating refined white flour products—from soft white bread sandwiches for lunch to pancakes on weekends and macaroni and cheese for dinner. White flour makes up many foods people eat every day such as pasta, muffins, bagels, buns, flour tortillas, pizza, pancakes, sandwiches, crackers, dinner rolls, bread sticks, cakes, doughnuts, and pastries. We give foods fancy names like French bread, panini, sourdough, and baguettes—but they're still made of white flour. All these foods rapidly turn to sugar in the bloodstream and can contribute to inflammation. Such foods can give a "doughboy look" to our faces by causing facial edema (a build up of fluid between cells) and puffiness under the eyes. Some of this is due to an allergic-type reaction, which can also contribute to dark circles under the eyes.

Identify and Avoid Food Allergens

Many food allergies and sensitivities (allergy-like reactions) raise levels of IgE (immunoglobulin E), which triggers an inflammatory response. Allergic reactions may be greatest in one part of the body, such as the nasal area, sinuses, or the gut, but activated immune cells migrate to other parts of the body and frequently attack healthy cells, causing a host of symptoms. In this heightened state of alert, other substances are released such as adrenaline and cortisol. These stressful changes add to wear and tear on the body and contribute to inflammation, which promotes wrinkles and other signs of aging. And it can also show up on the face in the form of puffiness and edema.

The most common food allergens are wheat, dairy, peanuts, corn, soy, sugar, and shellfish. Try avoiding these foods for a period of time to see if various physical symptoms clear up and your immune system becomes stronger. You may be surprised that certain foods are related to physical reactions that no one has ever been able to solve for you such as migraine headaches, sleep disturbances, depressed immunity, and skin problems such as rashes, bumps, acne, or rosacea (an inflammatory skin disorder characterized by redness and pimples).

If you think allergic reactions don't cause signs of aging, take a closer look at your face after you have one. Recently, I had an allergic reaction to something I ate that caused a full-blown migraine. I was really sick—from blinding headache to nausea—but for just a day this time (a good sign that my vitality is improving). I pinned down the cause: I'd eaten something breaded, forgetting that the breading was made of wheat. (I'm very sensitive to wheat.) Sitting in a restaurant the next day waiting for breakfast, my husband commented on new wrinkles around my eyes that weren't there a few days before. "That's inflammation at work," I said, "and it's time for a vegetable juice cleanse to flush them away."

Is it any wonder that many Americans can't lose weight, have blood sugar problems, experience insulin resistance, and age prematurely? For many, their entire day is filled with one high-carb, refined food after another and blood sugar that is bouncing around like a yo-yo.

If you want a more contoured face with less sags, bags, flabby skin, crinkly lines, and puffiness, a lean protein, low-carbohydrate diet (especially omitting refined carbs) that is rich in antioxidants and dominant in vegetables and other whole foods is the best fare.

Refined Carbohydrates to Avoid

Bagels	Flour tortillas
Baguettes	Muffins
Biscuits	Oatmeal (instant)
Bread	Pancakes
Bread sticks	Panini
Breakfast pastries	Pasta
Buns	Pizza dough
Cereals (packaged)	Rolls
Cereal bars	Sourdough
Crackers	Stuffing
Dinner rolls	Wheat tortillas
Doughnuts	White rice/puffed rice
English muffins	Rice cakes
French bread	Waffles

SUGAR AND SWEETS

Think wrinkles when you think sugar (and that includes all sweets) and avoid them like you would a root canal. Research indicates that higher amounts of sugar can raise triglycerides, LDL cholesterol, and insulin and lead to insulin resistance. Sweets can increase the number of wrinkles and contribute to a puffy, less-contoured face. And they can play a role in cancer, diabetes, and heart disease. Animal studies have shown that increased amounts of sucrose in the diet of rodents reduced their life span. Studies also show that diabetics who don't control blood sugar levels age much faster than those who do control it.

Blood sugar reacts with minerals such as iron and copper, creating free radicals, oxidized fat, and inflammation. Higher blood sugar also contributes to fat storage. And as previously discussed, foods that convert quickly to blood sugar can cause browning of the skin (from freckles to age spots) and a loss of the skin's elasticity.

Avoid sugar in all forms: white table sugar, brown sugar, powdered sugar, dehydrated sugarcane, fructose, dextrose, molasses, corn syrup, table syrup, as well as fruit juice and dried fruit. (Use natural sweeteners such as honey, pure maple syrup, brown rice syrup, and malt barley syrup sparingly.) When blood sugar spikes up, free radicals are created that oxidize fat, which includes LDL cholesterol. Oxidized LDL can contribute to plaque deposits in the lining of arteries. These simple and refined carbs may be some of the worst culprits when it comes to heart disease.

There's another reason to avoid sweets: Glucose that isn't stored as fat can attach to proteins in your body, which, similar to oxidation, impairs the performance of cells. This process is known as *glycation*. Glycation of proteins is a very unhealthy process, as it can produce what are called advanced glycated end products (AGEs). These altered proteins can build up in tissues, affecting cellular function and accelerating aging. Glycation damages protein to the extent that white blood cells will have to concentrate on gobbling them up, which puts a strain on your ability to repair the body and maintain a strong immunity level. And glycated proteins make a person very pro-inflammatory.

It is also wise to avoid *all* sugar substitutes such as aspartame (Equal or NutraSweet) and sucralose (Splenda) because of the negative reactions they can produce in the body. Most people choose sugar substitutes hoping to prevent weight gain and some people even say they'll chance the negative consequences because they can't afford to gain weight. But there is no scientific evidence proving that sugar substitutes prevent weight gain. Rather, they indicate the opposite.

A study published in the *International Journal of Obesity* looked at fourteen women who were given drinks of aspartame-sweetened lemonade, sucrose-sweetened lemonade, and carbonated mineral water on three separate days. The women ate significantly more food when they were given aspartame-sweetened beverages. Miryam Ehrlich Williamson, author of *Blood Sugar Blues,* says, "I know of people who were unable to lose weight, and some who actually gained, on a low-carbohydrate diet that included liberal use of sugar substitutes." There is also concern as to whether sugar substitutes can trigger insulin response. Williamson says her hunch is that some people are conditioned to pump insulin whenever they taste something sweet, just as Pavlov's dog learned to salivate when it heard a bell ring.

Aspartame

Aspartame is the most popular artificial sweetener. It is a chemical combination of the amino acids phenylalanine and aspartic acid. Current data collected from thousands of reports indicate that aspartame may contribute to headaches, mood changes, neurological disorders, seizures, and brain tumors.

Sucralose

Billed as the next generation of sugar substitutes, and marketed as a healthy sugar substitute, sucralose (popularly known as Splenda) is turning out to be anything but that. It is a noncaloric sweetener that is six hundred times sweeter than sucrose (white table sugar). Sucralose is created by chlorinating sugar (sucrose), which involves chemically changing the structure of the sugar molecule by substituting three chlorine atoms for three hydroxyl (oxygen and hydrogen) groups.

There are very few human studies regarding the safety of sucralose.

One study with diabetics reported an increase in glycosylated hemoglobin, which is the marker of long-term blood glucose. According to the FDA, "increases in glycosalation in hemoglobin imply lessening of [blood sugar] control in diabetics." Research with animals shows quite negative results: shrunken thymus gland, enlarged liver and kidneys, atrophy of lymph follicles in the spleen and thymus, reduced growth rate, decreased red blood cell count, hyperplasia of the pelvis, diarrhea, and a host of pregnancy problems. (For more information, see Dr. Joseph Mercola's article on sucralose at www.mercola.com/2000/dec/3/sucralose_dangers.htm.)

Blood sugar lows can cause carb cravings, and to prevent them, it's important to eat small healthy snacks mid-morning or afternoon to keep blood sugar stable. Be aware that sugar cravings can also be caused by a deficiency in the mineral chromium (a trace mineral) or a protein deficiency.

Avoiding sweets may be easier said than done since sugar is very addictive. When sugar cravings hit, substitute low-sugar fruit such as berries for a sweet or eat a protein snack like almonds or a slice of turkey breast that will help stabilize blood sugar. If you have strong urges to eat sweets or other carbs, supplement your diet with chromium and eat a protein snack in between meals. If the carb cravings persist, you may have a condition known as *Candida albicans,* which is an overgrowth of yeast in the body that causes cravings for sugar, alcohol, and carbs such as bread—preferred food for yeasts. It's also important to get rid of yeasts, because they are choice food for parasites. (Take the quiz on p. 234 to determine the likelihood.)

Sweets to Avoid

Barbecue sauce with sweetener
Brownies
Brown Sugar
Cakes
Candy
Cookies
Corn syrup/high-fructose
    corn syrup
Dehydrated sugarcane juice
Desserts
Dextrose
Energy bars (many energy bars
    contain too much sugar or
    alternative sweeteners)
Frozen yogurt
Fructose
Gelatin
Ice cream

Jams
Jellies
Ketchup
Molasses
Mousse
Pies
Powdered sugar
Pudding
Sorbet/frozen yogurt
Syrups
Sugar and sweeteners/all sugar
    substitutes
Table syrup, especially artificial
    syrup; use pure maple syrup in
    small amounts
Whipped topping
White table sugar

SWEETENERS TO LIMIT
(Use in small amounts)

Brown rice syrup and malt
    barley syrup (better than
    most; can be found at
    health food stores)
Honey
Pure maple syrup

ARTIFICIAL SWEETENERS
(Avoid)

Aspartame
Sucralose

SALT

The refined table salt most people are accustomed to using is highly processed and has had its minerals removed; what remains is primarily sodium chloride. Anticaking chemicals, potassium iodide, and dextrose (sugar) are then added to make table salt. Perhaps one of the reasons so many people tend to overeat salty foods is that their bodies are craving the minerals that have been refined away, which will never be satisfied by processed salt. One big reason to avoid overeating refined salt is that, in a similar manner to sugar, it can contribute to brown spots and freckling—known in Oriental medicine as "salt burns." The best choice is Celtic sea salt (see Chapter 2, p. 70).

FATS AND OILS

Fats, technically known as lipids, from animal and vegetable sources provide a concentrated source of energy. They are also the building blocks for cell membranes, hormones, and prostaglandins. If a lipid is liquid at room temperature, it is called *oil*. If it is solid, it is called *fat*.

A variety of lipids can be found in many food sources in nature: meat (such as tallow and lard), fish (fish oil), vegetables and fruits (corn, olive, avocado), nuts (walnut, macadamia, coconut), seeds (sesame, grape seed), legumes (peanut, soybean), and whole grains (wheat, rice, rye). In their whole form within the food, most are healthy fats and oils.

Unhealthy fats can be found in margarine and shortening (the partially hydrogenated oils), refined oils, and the very worst of all—oils that are heated to very high temperatures and used over and over again for deep-frying. Within this category are the most damaging fats—the *trans-fatty acids* (altered fats that are toxic). When oils are turned into margarine and shortening by partial hydrogenation, trans fats are created. Foods such as French fries, onion rings, and deep-fried shrimp are examples of foods that contain a lot of trans-fatty acids. Also, trans fats are used as a preservative in a host of baked goods and pancake mixes; they can even be found in peanut butter.

Trans fats are very detrimental to our health, contributing to heart disease, cancer, diabetes, obesity, low birth weight, and immune dysfunction. They disrupt cellular function and make cell membranes stiff and inflexible, which contributes to insulin resistance. They interfere with the conversion of omega-6 and omega-3 fatty acids to their most usable form in the body, resulting in essential fatty acid deficiency, which can show up in a host of skin problems such as eczema. They have been shown to lower the good HDL cholesterol, raise the bad LDL, and increase blood insulin. They can also cause a host of pregnancy and birth problems and precipitate childhood asthma. It is advisable to avoid trans-fatty acids completely.

The polyunsaturated oils such as corn, soy, and safflower that we've been told to consume because they are "heart healthy" have turned out to be anything but that. These double-bond fatty acids tend to polymerize, which means they easily bond with each other and with other molecules, and that's not good for your health or your skin. They have a great propensity to turn rancid (oxidize) in the body and when used for cooking or exposed to oxygen, moisture, or heat, they oxidize easily. Rancid oils generate more free radicals, which are very reactive and attack cell walls contributing to damaged skin, wrinkles, sagging skin, and other signs of aging. Heart disease was a rare thing prior to the introduction of refined vegetable oils into the diet. Retrospective studies show increased cardiovascular risk from diets high in polyunsaturated oils.

The typical American diet contains from 10 to 30 percent fat from polyunsaturated fatty acids in the form of commercial vegetable oils. Most of these polyunsaturated oils are abundant in omega-6 linoleic acid, with very little of the healthy linolenic acid (an omega-3). A diet with excess omega-6s, along with too few omega-3s, can result in inflammation, depressed immunity, and weight gain.

Many polyunsaturated vegetable oils can also contribute to a process known as glycation. Glycation in the food industry is known as caramelization (caramelizing means browning). As this process continues, we age faster because the fatty acids in our body, especially the polyunsaturated fatty acids, turn rancid, or glycate (turn brown).

To avoid these effects, refined vegetable oils such as safflower, sunflower, canola, corn, and soy oil should be completely eliminated from the diet. And, be sure to avoid all fake fats such as olestra as well. The best oils to use for food preparation are extra-virgin olive oil and coconut oil.

Fats and Oils to Avoid

Canola

Corn

Fake fats such as olestra

Margarine

Polyunsaturated oils (including
   commercial salad dressings
   made with oils listed at right)

Safflower

Shortening

Soybean

Sunflower

DAIRY PRODUCTS

It's best to limit dairy products as much as possible. Many people are lactose intolerant or allergic to dairy. Lactose intolerance is the rule rather than the exception among many peoples of the world, particularly Native American, Mediterranean, Asian, African, and Middle Eastern peoples. Also, lactose intolerance becomes more prevalent as we age. (A dairy allergy is different from lactose intolerance in that it is caused by an immune reaction to the protein in milk.) Ingesting allergens and foods to which we're intolerant increases inflammation, which contributes to wrinkles, puffiness, facial edema, and dark circles under the eyes. Also, referring back to the study on the foods that contributed most to skin damage, full-fat milk was implicated as one of the contributors. (See Chapter 2, p. 33.)

Dairy Products to Limit or Avoid

Avoid all high-fat dairy products as much as possible, especially these:

High-fat cheeses such as cheddar, Muenster, Brie, cream cheese, and
    especially cheeses that are processed (choose only natural cheeses)
Ice cream
Milk and cream
Sweetened yogurt and frozen yogurt

ANIMAL PROTEINS

Red meat and animal fats should be limited in the diet. Toxins tend to be stored in the fat more than the muscle. Also, full-fat milk and other high-fat dairy products and red meat are among the foods associated with the most skin damage in the study discussed earlier (see p. 33). To avoid inflammatory responses, it is wise to limit red meat (beef, veal, buffalo, lamb, pork) to no more than one serving per week.

Animal Proteins to Limit or Avoid

Beef in general should be limited, but especially avoid fatty cuts (more toxins are stored in fat than muscle):

Bacon

Brisket

Honey-baked ham

Liver

Liverwurst

Pork

Processed poultry products

Rib eye steak

Ribs

BEVERAGES

Coffee, black tea, chocolate, and sodas are loaded with caffeine (and sodas and chocolate with sugar or sugar substitutes as well), which taxes the adrenal glands and raises cortisol and insulin. In addition to affecting aging, these beverages also promote storage of fat, particularly on the midsection. If you need a little caffeine lift, choose green tea. It has some caffeine, but only about one third that of a cup of coffee. Its nutritional rating is excellent and it contributes to cancer prevention and antiaging. Green tea comes in decaffeinated varieties for those who want no caffeine. Herbal teas are also excellent choices and can be iced or served hot.

Avoid soda pop and diet sodas. These beverages are loaded with chemicals and sugar, and diet sodas with sugar substitutes. Because of the chemicals and sugars, sodas add to the body's toxic load and contribute to inflammation; the sweeteners lead to sugar imbalances and ultimately insulin resistance. Also, avoid powdered drink mixes. And limit fruit juice to small amounts; they contain too much fruit sugar.

Alcohol interferes with efficient circulation of blood to the skin, which transports nutrients for healing and repair. It also acts similar to sugar in the body, increasing insulin secretion, which can cause spikes and dips in blood sugar levels that contribute to blood sugar imbalances and insulin resistance. It also causes inflammation due to aldehydes, which are metabolites of alcohol that play a part in damage of cell plasma membranes.

Beverages to Greatly Limit or Avoid

Alcohol: beer, wine, liquor, cordials (liqueurs)

Anything with sugar substitutes or sweeteners

Black tea

Chocolate drinks/cocoa

Coffee

Fruit juice, especially bottled and canned

Soda pop/ diet sodas

Sports drinks

PROCESSED FOODS

Chemicals are detrimental to our health and harmful to our appearance. These substances create "toxic sludge" in the body that collects in the spaces between cells (interstitial spaces), and in tissues and organs causing inflammation, cellular oxidation, and widespread toxicity. Poor elimination of wastes can contribute to facial puffiness, water retention (edema), and cellulite on the hips, thighs, and buttocks, which are pockets of water, toxins, and fat held in place by hardened connective tissue. It is believed that toxins cause the water to be held in these pockets, contributing to the orange peel look. If left in the body for a long time, toxins can lead to cancer. This is one of the reasons I recommend cleansing the body periodically and a primary reason I wrote *The Complete Cancer Cleanse*.

Snack foods, processed foods, and many packaged foods are sources of chemicals—additives, fillers, preservatives, trans-fatty acids, dyes, flavor enhancers, heavy metals such as mercury, aluminum, and cadmium, nitrites, nitrates, leavening, firming agents, and dough conditioners. Foods sprayed with pesticides, herbicides, and fungicides, and grown with chemical fertilizers also add to the body's toxic load. (It's healthiest to buy organically grown food whenever possible.) Read all labels. A good rule to remember is: If you can't pronounce it, don't buy it.

Processed Foods/Snack Foods to Avoid

It is not possible to list all snack and processed foods. If the product comes in a package, carton, can, or box, always read the label and avoid anything with additives.

Chips: tortilla, potato, corn

Cheese snacks

Crackers

Dips

Energy bars and drinks (some contain chemicals)

Frozen dinners

Pretzels

Soups: dried or canned

Soy crisps and snacks

TOBACCO

The joke about smokers' wrinkled-looking "prune lips" is not a joke for those who have them. There are very few things that could be more damaging to the skin than smoking. Tobacco smoke is known to decrease vitamin C levels and increase toxicity. Vitamin C is a necessary cofactor for the production of collagen, which maintains the elasticity of the skin and gives it firmness and contour. Cigarette (also pipe and cigar) smoke is loaded with free radicals and contains high amounts of cadmium (a metallic element that is toxic). These toxic substances attack proteins and fats and cause damaged cells, which cause cross-linking of proteins (collagen and elastin) to other molecules. As collagen hardens and elastin tissue diminishes, skin becomes less flexible—more leathery and wrinkled, puckered, and creased.

4

Step 1:
The Quick Start Programs

The quick cleanses of Step 1 begin with either an all-day vegetable juice fast or a two-day raw-food rejuvenator, both of which will enliven your body and help repair damaged cells. Actually you don't have to pick and choose—you can use both of these programs for a spectacular kickoff to your Wrinkle Cleanse program or to follow up the 14-Day Wrinkle Cleanse Diet in Chapter 5—whichever you wish. With these programs, you should see immediate results in your appearance—more vibrant, glowing skin and sparkling eyes. You may notice that you look more rested and refreshed. And, you may experience an increase in energy. You can return to these programs at any time whenever you need to recharge your Wrinkle Cleanse program, prepare for a special event, or cleanse your body when you've overindulged.

The advantages of a one-day vegetable juice fast are cleansing and elimination of wastes and toxins and rejuvenation of tired, sluggish cells.

This fast day gives the digestive organs such as the stomach, intestines, pancreas, gallbladder, and liver a chance to rest and focus on cleansing and repair. During a fast, every cell has a chance to catch up on important work, because there are fewer demands placed on them. They can focus on repair and clearing out waste, like you can focus on sweeping the floor or repairing a broken door when you have a day off.

The two-day raw-food rejuvenator offers light detoxification and a chance to feed your body power-packed, energizing nutrients. The enzymes in raw foods assist your digestive organs so they don't have to work as hard. And the antioxidants, minerals, and other nutrients in raw foods feed your cells optimal nutrition. Many people say that after a raw-food regimen, their skin glows, hair shines, and eyes sparkle with new life.

You may want to try both of these quick-start cleanses right away, in which case, start with the two-day raw-food rejuvenator, which will prepare your body for the one-day vegetable juice fast.

Benefits of Fasting

Cleansing (detoxification)

Rejuvenation

Revitalization

Clearer skin/improved skin color and tone

Clearer whites of eyes

Lessening of wrinkles and lines

Skin tightening

Improved vision, hearing, taste, and smell

Weight loss

Increased energy

Improved sleep

Improvement in mood/better attitude

Increased mental clarity

When you fast, consider adding cleansing boosters such as colonics (see p. 139 for more information), probiotics (good bacteria to replenish healthy bacteria, vitamin C, and other antioxidants; see Chapter 7). Also, relaxation techniques such as massage, sauna (especially far-infrared sauna), aromatherapy baths, deep breathing gentle exercise, walking, and meditation or prayer are very beneficial.

THE ONE-DAY VEGETABLE JUICE FAST

The one-day vegetable juice cleanse is an all-liquid day that helps rejuvenate your entire body. It's easiest to choose a weekend day or any other day when you don't have to work outside your home, but if that's not possible, it's easy enough to take juices to work in a thermos. During that day you will drink only vegetable juices (a little low-sugar fruit juice is permitted), water, sparkling mineral water, warm vegetable broth, and herbal or green teas. That's all. This cleansing day is a great boost to antiaging and will especially help you get rid of excess stored water, mucus, and toxins. It helps to rejuvenate the body at the cellular level. And it provides an abundance of antioxidants to neutralize free radicals and help your body repair damaged cells.

You can kick off your Wrinkle Cleanse program with this one-day fast, or you can add it as the fifteenth day, after your two weeks of the Wrinkle Cleanse Diet. You may also extend the juice fast for a second day, making it a weekend cleanse. Some people like to fast one day a week, as do my husband and I, and you can do that during the 14-Day Wrinkle Cleanse Diet. This is your program and you can tailor it to fit your desires.

If you have a special event coming up and you want to lose a pound or two and look especially vibrant and rejuvenated, this one-day cleanse can make a big difference in how you look and feel. Even if you have to work outside the home, you can plan ahead and make your fast happen without stress so you're refreshed for your special event. The juice fast is also excellent to flush out toxins and waste if you have overindulged in foods and beverages that are not part of the Wrinkle Cleanse program while on vacation, at a special event, or during a time of stress.

THE ONE-DAY JUICE FAST MENU

The Evening Before
The evening meal before your juice fast should be light and preferably just a green salad with a variety of raw vegetables and a simple dressing of lemon juice, olive oil, and herbs.

Breakfast
7:00 a.m. or upon rising: Herbal or green tea with lemon juice or hot water with lemon and a dash of cayenne pepper
7:30 a.m.: Morning Energy Cocktail (p. 95) or vegetable or low-sugar fruit juice of choice

Mid-morning
9:00 a.m.: 8 ounces of water or herbal tea
10:00 a.m.: Vegetable juice of choice
11:00 a.m.: 8 ounces of water or sparkling mineral water with lemon or vitamin C powder in water*

Lunch
Noon: Spicy Tomato on Ice (p. 96), V-8 juice, or vegetable juice of choice

Mid-afternoon

1:30 p.m.: 8 ounces water or sparkling mineral water with lemon

2:30 p.m.: 8 ounces water or sparkling mineral water with lemon or vitamin C powder

3:00 p.m.: Warm vegetable broth or vegetable juice of choice

4:00 p.m.: 8 ounces water or sparkling mineral water with lemon

5:00 p.m.: 8 ounces water or sparkling mineral water with lemon

Dinner

6:00 p.m.: 8–10 ounces of vegetable juice of choice *or* Cold Cucumber Avocado Soup (p. 97) or Cold Carrot Avocado Soup (p. 98)

(You may also add a cup of warm vegetable broth.)

---

*Sparkling mineral water may be substituted for water at any time. You may add a squeeze of lemon or lime for added flavor, or a teaspoon of unsweetened cranberry or black cherry juice concentrate, which you can find at many health food stores. Also, vitamin C powder (buffered ascorbic acid) is excellent is assisting the cleansing process; as an antioxidant it binds with free radicals and neutralizes them. You can either mix it with water or juice or use Emer'gen-C Lite (this is the brand name for a powdered vitamin C, which has less sweetener and contains seven minerals including sulfur, found at health food stores).

Juices for Specific Cleansing

These juice recommendations are based on Paavo Airola's *How to Get Well*, Norman Walker's *Fresh Vegetable and Fruit Juices*, and my own *The Juice Lady's Guide to Juicing for Health*.

FRUIT
Lemon: liver, gallbladder
Apple: liver, intestines
Pear: gallbladder
Papaya: stomach
Black cherry: colon

VEGETABLES
Carrot: bladder, liver

Beets: bladder, liver

Beet greens: gallbladder, liver

Cucumber: bladder, liver

Greens: skin, liver

Celery: kidneys

Radish: liver (also good for the thyroid)

Comfrey: intestines

Spinach: bladder, liver

Parsley: kidneys, liver

Wheatgrass: liver, gallbladder

RECIPES FOR THE ONE-DAY
VEGETABLE JUICE FAST

Morning Energy Cocktail

If you think vegetable juice is going to present a taste challenge, try this recipe. It's delicious and loaded with antioxidants. This juice combo has about 18 carbohydrates, and it's a good carb-investment, considering it's replete with antioxidants, soluble fiber, enzymes, phytochemicals, minerals, and especially the antiaging nutrients alpha- and beta-carotene.

1 cucumber, peeled if not organic	½ beet with leaves
½ lemon, peeled	2 stalks celery
1 or 2 carrots, scrubbed	Handful fresh parsley
	1-inch piece fresh ginger root

1. Cut the cucumber in half and push half the cucumber through the juicer. Follow with the remaining ingredients and end with the other half of the cucumber.
2. Stir and drink as soon as possible.

Serves 1

Nutritional analysis (per 1 carrot): 207 calories (7.8% from fat) • 2g fat • 8g protein • 18g carbohydrate • >2g dietary fiber • 0mg cholesterol • 173mg sodium

Spicy Tomato on Ice

This is a refreshing drink especially in the afternoon, but good any time of day, and it has only 9 carbs.

> 1 vine-ripened tomato
> 1 cucumber, peeled if not organic
> 2 stalks celery
> Dash of hot sauce
> Ice cubes (optional)

1. Cut the tomato into chunks that will fit your juicer and cut the cucumber in half lengthwise.
2. Juice the tomato, cucumber, and celery.
3. Add a dash of hot sauce to taste and stir. Serve over ice, if desired.
   Serves 1

Nutritional analysis (per serving): 39 calories (9.9% from fat) • 1g fat • 2g protein • 9g carbohydrate • >2g dietary fiber • 0mg cholesterol • 96mg sodium

Cold Cucumber Avocado Soup

This is a delicious, satisfying cold soup with the added beneficial fats from the avocado.

1½ cups fresh cucumber juice (about 2 cucumbers)
¼ cup fresh lemon juice
1 tablespoon chopped green onions
1 tablespoon chopped red onion
1 tablespoon chopped fresh parsley
1 large ripe avocado, peeled and seeded

1 large or 2 medium garlic cloves, minced
3 small sprigs fresh basil, chopped (optional)
1 teaspoon tamari or light soy sauce
1 to 2 teaspoons curry powder, or to taste
½ teaspoon ground cumin

1. Combine the juice and all other ingredients in a blender and puree until smooth. If the soup is a bit thick, you may add a little more cucumber juice or lemon juice.
2. Pour the soup into bowls and serve cold. You may garnish with fresh basil or any other fresh herbs of choice.

Serves 2

Nutritional analysis (per serving): 186 calories (68.9% from fat) • 16g fat • 3g protein • 13g carbohydrate • 4g dietary fiber • 0mg cholesterol • 182mg sodium

Cold Carrot Avocado Soup

～～～

This soup is very energizing and is loaded with alpha- and beta-carotene.

1 cup fresh carrot juice (6 to 8 carrots)
1 avocado, peeled and seeded
Dash of cumin

Combine all the ingredients in a blender and process until smooth. Chill and serve.

Serves 1

Nutritional analysis (per serving): 415 calories (62% from fat) • 31g fat • 6g protein • 36g carbohydrate • 7g dietary fiber • 0mg cholesterol • 86mg sodium

Vegetable Broth

～～～

You can easily make your own vegetable broth, which is much healthier than the canned version. This broth is rich in minerals.

½ cup chopped onions
½ cup chopped celery
½ cup chopped carrots
½ cup fresh parsley

½ cup chopped turnips
½ cup chopped parsnips
1 or 2 leaves kale
Pinch sea salt or Celtic salt

Add all ingredients to a pot and add enough cold water to cover and simmer for about 1½ hours, or until vegetables are tender. Strain the broth off of the vegetables and use the vegetables for composting or other uses; chill the broth. Heat a cup of the broth at a time, as desired.

Makes 5 to 6 servings

Nutritional analysis per serving (estimated): 20 calories (31% from fat) • 1g fat • 2g protein • 3g carbohydrate • 0g dietary fiber • 0mg cholesterol • 300–500mg sodium

A Note About Fasting

Fasting is abstaining from certain types of foods. Juice fasting is abstaining from all solid foods and consuming only juices made from fruits and vegetables, along with plenty of water, vegetable broth, and herbal teas for a designated period of time. Fresh juices are excellent for cleansing because they are easily digested and are replete with enzymes, vitamins, and minerals.

Fasting dates back thousands of years. The Essenes, a Jewish sect that existed around the time of Christ, espoused fasting to purify the body and heighten communion with God. Scriptures tell us that Jesus fasted. Gandhi, Plato, and Socrates fasted. Nearly every religion encourages fasting as a spiritual discipline. Norman Cousins, known for his laugh therapy to regain health, also taught on fasting for health and healing and fasted himself.

Unless people fast, they usually carry the toxic burden of chemicals such as PCBs and DDT for a lifetime. When you fast, chemicals are mobilized. Fasting increases the cleansing process and releases toxins from the intestines, kidneys, bladder, liver, lungs, and skin. It is not recommended that you fast for more than five days without professional supervision, and that you not perform water fasting unless you have fasted before with vegetable juices and eaten a healthy diet. Too many toxins are released during water fasting, and without the benefit of antioxidants to neutralize them, they can cause more damage than good experienced by their mobilization. (Fasting is not recommended for children under the age of eighteen or for pregnant or lactating women.)

Elson Haas, MD, author of *Staying Healthy with Nutrition,* says, "Much of aging and disease . . . results from 'biochemical suffocation' where our cells do not get enough oxygen and nutrients or cannot adequately eliminate wastes. Fasting helps us to decrease this suffocation by allowing the cells to eliminate and clear the old products. Fasting is like turning off and cleaning a complex and valuable machine so that it will function better and longer." Fasting generates a discharge of toxic material and waste matter such as mucus and chemicals from the gastrointestinal and respiratory tracts, and the sinuses and restores cellular function. This is key in restoring one's youthful bloom and a major part of the Wrinkle Cleanse program.

In his book *Triumph over Disease,* Jack Goldstein, DPM, tells his true story of overcoming ulcerative colitis by water fasting and a vegetarian diet. He tested his tongue, urine, feces, and perspiration to determine the effectiveness and found that "the contents [during a fast] are different than normal—that toxins like DDT do get removed."

Years ago I, too, discovered the healing benefits of fasting, which I outline in my book *The Juice Lady's Guide to Juicing for Health.* I suffered from chronic fatigue syndrome (CFS) that was debilitating. I had to quit an exciting job, because I was too sick to work. With no hope, other than my self-designed cleanse programs, I embarked on a five-day vegetable juice fast and then periodic juice fasts combined with a vegetarian diet for three months. At the end, I was completely well.

THE TWO-DAY RAW-FOOD REJUVENATOR

This two-day, raw-food diet is very energizing and revitalizing. If you want to look a bit younger and more vibrant and shed a pound or two quickly for any occasion, then try this raw-food plan. It can transform your face as well as your health in a short time. Or you may want to kickoff your Wrinkle Cleanse program with this two-day plan, followed by the one-day vegetable juice fast. You can also use this plan to follow the 14-Day Wrinkle Cleanse Diet.

For two days you will eat only raw foods—nothing cooked. That's right, all your meals will be raw fruits, vegetables, sea vegetables (soaked to rehydrate), sprouts, herbs, seeds, and nuts. You may also have dehydrated crackers that have not been heated over 118°F. You may extend this diet to three days or more (some people eat a mostly raw-food diet year round) or make 50 to 75 percent of your diet raw food, depending on your needs, the time of year, and how you feel on the diet. You may use any raw-food recipes you like for your meals, but if you decide to go raw for more than a couple of days, a good raw-foods recipe book would be very helpful.

TWO-DAY RAW-FOOD REJUVENATOR MENU

DAY 1

Breakfast

7:00 a.m. or upon rising: Herbal tea, green tea, or hot water and lemon with a dash of cayenne

7:30–8:00 a.m.: Fresh vegetable juice of choice

Sliced tomatoes and avocado sprinkled with sea salt and chopped herbs

Mid-morning

9:00 a.m.: 8 ounces of water or herbal tea

9:30 a.m.: 8 ounces of water

10:30 a.m.: Herbal tea, green tea, or vegetable juice with vegetable sticks

11:00 a.m.: 8 ounces of water

11:30 a.m.: 8 ounces of water or sparkling mineral water with lemon

Lunch

Noon: Large green salad with lots of vegetables and sprouts and fresh salsa or lemon juice for dressing

Mid-afternoon

1:30 p.m.: 8 ounces water

2:30 p.m.: 8 ounces water or sparkling mineral water with lemon

3:00 p.m.: Herbal tea, green tea, warm vegetable broth, or vegetable juice with sprouts or raw nuts or seeds

4:00 p.m.: 8 ounces water

5:00 p.m.: 8 ounces water or sparkling mineral water with lemon

Dinner

6:00 p.m.: 8–10 ounces of vegetable juice of choice or Cold Cucumber Avocado Soup (p. 97) or Cold Carrot Avocado Soup (p. 98)

Sprout salad: Use a variety of sprouts mixed with greens and fresh salsa or lemon juice for dressing

DAY 2

Breakfast

7:00 a.m. or upon rising: Herbal tea, green tea, or hot water and lemon with a dash of cayenne

7:30–8:00 a.m.: Very Berry Smoothie (made without dairy) (p. 179)

Mid-morning

9:00 a.m.: 8 ounces of water

9:30 a.m.: 8 ounces of water

10:30 a.m.: Herbal tea, green tea, or vegetable juice with vegetable sticks

11:00 a.m.: 8 ounces of water

11:30 a.m.: 8 ounces of water or sparkling mineral water with lemon

Lunch

Noon: Gazpacho soup (p. 192)

Green salad with sprouts and fresh salsa or lemon juice for
  dressing

Mid-afternoon

1:30 p.m.: 8 ounces water

2:30 p.m.: 8 ounces water

3:00 p.m.: Herbal tea, green tea, warm vegetable broth, or vegetable juice and sprouts or raw nuts or seeds

4:00 p.m.: 8 ounces water

5:00 p.m.: 8 ounces water or sparkling mineral water with lemon

Dinner

6:00 p.m.: 8–10 ounces of vegetable juice of choice

Cold raw vegetable plate with fresh salsa or lemon juice for
  dressing

RECIPE FOR A COOL-WEATHER CLEANSE

Autumn Rejuvenation Soup

During the cooler days of autumn and winter, you may not be able to
embark on an all-raw diet or juice fast. The autumn rejuvenation soup
along with the warm vegetable broth, herbal teas, and some juice may

be just the thing your body needs. Follow the two-day raw-food rejuvenator and substitute this soup for your lunch or dinner.

3 cups purified water	¼ cup chopped cilantro
1 tablespoon ginger root, minced	¼ cup chopped parsley
	1 teaspoon extra-virgin olive oil
1 to 2 tablespoons miso paste	Juice of ½ lemon
1 to 2 green onions, chopped	Pinch of cayenne pepper

In a medium pan, bring the water to a boil, add the ginger root, and simmer for 10 minutes. Stir in the miso paste to taste. Turn off the heat, add all the other ingredients, and steep for 10 minutes. Serve warm.

Serves 2

Nutritional analysis: 70 calories (40% from fat) • 3.4g fat • 2.5g protein • 2g fiber • 9g carbohydrate • 0mg cholesterol • 480mg sodium

THE NEXT STEP

Having completed the one-day vegetable juice fast and the two-day raw-food rejuvenator, you are ready for Step 2—the exciting 14-Day Wrinkle Cleanse Diet. (Or, if these days followed the 14-Day Diet, then go to the Cleanses.) This diet is designed to help you change your way of eating and adopt a new, healthy plan for life. The dietary program can help you restore collagen, improve your facial tone, restore elasticity and tautness, and soften lines and wrinkles. This is the plan that will also help your body heal from ailments and prevent illnesses and chronic conditions in the future.

5

Step 2: The 14-Day Wrinkle Cleanse Diet

If you have completed Step 1, you should feel and look more refreshed and revitalized and be ready for Step 2. Or, you may be waiting to try Step 1 after you've completed the 14-Day Wrinkle Cleanse Diet. Either way, you're about to discover a new way of eating to create a younger-looking you. In two weeks you should look and feel healthier and more vibrant than you have in a while, perhaps a long while. If you have been protein deficient because your diet was focused on carbs, especially refined carbs and high-carb foods, you should notice your skin tightening and wrinkles softening. The nutrients provided by this diet will feed your collagen, which gives your skin support and helps it appear firmer. Your color and facial muscle tone should improve. And you should look more radiant and alive!

Step 2 of the Wrinkle Cleanse program introduces a low-carbohydrate diet, including plenty of vegetables, sprouts, vegetable juices, low-sugar fruit, whole grains, legumes, and lean proteins, while cutting calorie intake overall. It also encourages drinking eight to ten 8-ounce glasses of water each day. It eliminates white flour products, most starches, alcohol, sweeteners, sugar substitutes, coffee, and all junk food. These are the substances that increase inflammation and cause insulin resistance, cell oxidation, and visible signs of aging. There's lots of variety so you shouldn't miss the pizza, pasta, or bagels. Healthy fats, which include extra-virgin olive oil and virgin coconut oil, are incorporated into food preparation. (Coconut oil helps many people curb their cravings for sweets—an added bonus!) You shouldn't miss candy and desserts—those nasty little carbs that wreak havoc on your face, because cravings should soon disappear.

The menu plan with recipes will help you incorporate the Wrinkle Cleanse Diet into your daily life. Remember, this is just a guide. You can pick and choose what fits for you each day of the week and tailor the plan to fit your needs.

If you're ready to renew your face and your entire body, then you're ready to begin the 14-Day Wrinkle Cleanse Diet.

CUT CALORIES—EXTEND YOUR LIFE

Want to extend your life, experience a better quality of life right now, and look younger? Cut your calories, say the experts. According to the Harvard Medical School, calorie restriction has been shown to increase longevity in organisms ranging from yeasts to mammals. Controlled calorie intake is the only regimen that has been shown in laboratory tests thus far to increase life span. Numerous studies have shown that reducing calories may slow down aging, reduce age-related degenerative diseases, and increase longevity by reducing oxidative stress and cellular damage, promoting insulin sensitivity, and producing anti-inflammatory effects. Yes, all that—just by eating less food.

Perhaps the largest body of research to date on antiaging has to do with eating less. We know that calorie restriction reduces metabolic rate, promotes glucose and insulin regulation, reduces oxidative stress, and alters neuroendocrine and sympathetic nervous system function in animals.

Recently, researchers at the National Institute of Aging published a study in *Science* that linked three factors to longevity with calorie restriction in monkeys—lower body temperatures and insulin levels and high levels of DHEAs (natural steroid hormones). The calorie-restricted monkeys lived longer than their normally fed peers. In a human population study, researchers examined participant data from the Baltimore Longitudinal Study of Aging and found similar effects related to longevity in men. Though calories were not restricted with the men in the study, the same three factors were measured. The men with lower body temperature and insulin levels and higher levels of DHEAs lived longer than the men in the other half of the population studied.

Following the recommendations of the Food Guide Pyramid, Americans will eat between 2,000 and 2,500 calories per day. For an adult, a calorie-restricted diet would cut calories about 30 percent to somewhere between 1,400 and 1,700 calories a day.

When considering fewer calories, we need to make sure that we get high-nutrient content in the foods we choose, because, though we want to achieve calorie restriction, we don't want malnutrition. Calorie restriction is very different from rigid dieting or starvation, which is detrimental to one's health and will promote aging and have negative effects on metabolism, often causing weight gain. We want to choose a diet that contains all the necessary nutrients to support optimal health, and this means we can't afford empty calories such as those found in processed and refined foods.

Diets based on an abundance of fresh vegetables, vegetable juices, fruits, sprouts, legumes, nuts, seeds, whole grains, small amounts of healthy fats, sensible portions of lean animal protein (four to six ounces), and limited dairy products will be lower in calories. There's no room for junk food in a calorie-restricted diet designed to promote health and longevity.

Dr. Norman Walker, author of *Become Younger* and one of the pioneers of the raw food and fresh juice movement, was a shining example of the results of cutting calories. He ate a predominantly raw-foods diet with generous amounts of vegetables and vegetable juices. Though he didn't report the number of calories he ate daily, he did report on his healthy fruit and vegetable diet, which was obviously lower in calories than what the average American eats. He lived to be well over one hundred years of age in good health and looking much younger than his years.

Eating smaller meals more often throughout the day will keep your blood sugar stable and prevent big spikes and dips in blood sugar levels. This should help in preventing a food-binge in the evening—a time when blood sugar is often quite low, causing us to feel starved and sending us running for the chips when we walk in the front door. The evening meal is often when we tend to eat the most calories, which certainly doesn't contribute to a longer life and really packs on the weight, since we don't have much time to burn up what we eat in the evening.

Choosing nutrient-dense foods, such as those recommended in this program, will help to stabilize blood sugar and curb cravings for sweets, refined carbs, and salty junk food. Also, eating lighter for your evening meal and not eating after 7:30 p.m. will give your elimination organs a chance to do the work of cleansing and help you sleep better—a big boon for living a longer, healthier life.

THE 14-DAY MENU PLAN

The 14-Day Wrinkle Cleanse Diet includes healthy breakfasts, lunches, dinners, and snacks. Starting your day with a healthy breakfast is as important as ending it with a nutritious meal. When you start with a healthy breakfast, you're far less likely to be tempted by a doughnut or bagel and coffee for mid-morning break. A nutritious mid-morning snack and a healthy lunch will keep your blood sugar stable so you won't crash mid-afternoon and run for a candy bar and a latte. And a light, healthy dinner is the best way to end the day.

Strive to include raw foods with every meal, whether it's freshly made vegetable juice, sliced tomatoes or avocado, fresh berries, sprouts, raw nuts, or seeds. Include four to five servings of vegetables (one cup equals a serving) each day, two servings of fruit, and one or two servings of whole grains. Keep animal protein such as fish, chicken, or red meat serving sizes to around four to six ounces; soup, one to two cups. And though calorie counting is not a suggested part of this program, if you are prone to counting calories, strive for somewhere between 1,500 and 2,000 calories, keeping in mind that cutting calories can lengthen your life span.

Creating Healthy Meals

BREAKFAST
A healthy breakfast can be a glass of vegetable juice and some veggie sticks, or a protein-rich smoothie, whole grain cereal with fresh berries, eggs, or broiled fish. The important thing is that you eat a whole foods breakfast.

LUNCH

Lunch can be healthy soup and salad, a bean dish, a main course salad, broiled fish or baked chicken with greens, or a healthy turkey burger (no buns).

DINNER

A main course salad; steamed vegetables and brown rice; baked fish, turkey, or chicken; hearty soup and salad; or a vegetarian entrée with salad can make a healthy dinner.

SNACKS

Mid-morning and afternoon snacks help to keep your blood sugar stable. Choose from raw nuts, seeds, vegetable sticks, vegetable juice, smoothie, or fresh fruit.

BEVERAGES

For beverages, you have several choices: hot lemon water, iced or hot herbal tea, sparkling mineral water with lemon, lime, or a dash of cranberry or black cherry juice concentrate, and vegetable juice with small amounts of fruit juice for flavor, as desired. You'll also need to include eight to ten 8-ounce glasses of water each day to adequately hydrate your body.

The menu plan in this chapter and the recipes in Chapter 8 are designed to minimize inflammation, balance blood sugar, and provide the protein, fats, carbohydrates, enzymes, vitamins, and minerals that help slow down the aging process. You can choose any entrée you like for any meal and what appeals to you and works best for your lifestyle.

The Beauty of Raw Food

The typical American diet is very deficient in raw food—raw vegetables, fruit, sprouts, salad greens, nuts, and seeds. It's these foods, however, that are the great antiaging beautifiers. We need to eat more of them. Strive to make at least 50 percent of your diet raw. And watch your body transform.

Dr. Norman Walker tells a story in his book *Become Younger* of a thirty-one-year-old woman who was old before her time—aches, pains, low-energy, brain fog—and she looked about ten years older than her age. A friend, who had turned her own health around and erased a bundle of years off her face, persuaded this young woman to adopt a new diet. With nothing to lose, she cut out starches, sugar, red meat, milk, coffee, and black tea. Instead of soda pop, she daily drank one pint of freshly made vegetable juice. She included lots of salads and fresh fruit into her menu plan. Within a couple of months of making these changes, her work as a stenographer was so improved, she received a promotion. Prior to making the dietary changes, she did not date; she was considered plain and dull. Within a year of her diet revolution, she married her boss. Ten years later, in her early forties, she looked like she was in her late twenties.

If you want to become younger and more vibrant, eat more raw foods. And like the young woman in Dr. Walker's story, you may experience more benefits than just a younger-looking face.

14-DAY WRINKLE CLEANSE DIET MENU

DAY 1

Breakfast
Vegetable juice
Herbal tea with lemon or hot water and lemon
Green Chili Egg Scramble (p. 181)
Fresh sliced tomatoes with oregano

Mid-morning snack
Hot or iced herbal tea
Veggie sticks with Hummus, commercial or homemade (p. 204)

Lunch
Soup of choice
Spring greens with Lemon–Olive Oil Dressing (p. 201)
Low-sodium V-8 juice or Garden Cocktail (p. 176)

Mid-afternoon snack
10 raw almonds
Herbal iced tea with lemon

Dinner
Basic Garden Salad (p. 193) with Lemon-Tarragon Dressing
    (p. 201) or dressing of choice
Spicy Turkey Tostadas (p. 205)
Herbal tea with lemon

DAY 2

Breakfast
Very Berry Smoothie (p. 179) or Strawberry-Coconut Smoothie
(p. 180)

Mid-morning snack
¼ cup raw pumpkin or sunflower seeds
Hot or iced herbal tea

Lunch
Basic Garden Salad (p. 193) with Lemon-Tarragon Dressing
(p. 201)
French Tomato-Basil Soup (p. 186)

Mid-afternoon snack
Fresh vegetable juice of choice

Dinner
Basic Garden Salad (p. 193) with Basil-Parmesan Vinaigrette
(p. 202) or your favorite dressing
Gingered Beets with Sesame (p. 221)
Baked Tilapia with Tarragon-Quinoa Stuffing (p. 206)

DAY 3

Breakfast
Fresh vegetable juice
Broiled or smoked salmon
Vegetable sticks, sliced tomatoes, or ½ avocado

Mid-morning snack
4 celery sticks stuffed with almond butter

Lunch
Mushroom-Barley Soup (p. 187)
Sliced tomatoes with extra-virgin olive oil and balsamic vinegar

Mid-afternoon snack
6 raw almonds
Hot or iced herbal tea

Dinner
Coleslaw
Grilled Mustard-Rosemary Chicken (p. 208)
Steamed broccoli and carrots, sprinkled with lemon juice before
    serving

Dessert
1 cup fresh or frozen berries

DAY 4

Breakfast
Fresh vegetable juice
Oatmeal (not instant), amaranth, or quinoa, without sugar (you
    may use a healthful, low-carb sweetener)
Almond or rice milk
Fresh or frozen berries: blueberries, blackberries, or strawberries
¼ cup chopped nuts: almonds, pecans, or walnuts

Mid-morning snack
¼ cup raw sunflower seeds
Hot or iced herbal tea

Lunch
Grilled Salmon (p. 213) over salad greens with Lemon–Olive Oil
  Dressing (p. 201)

Mid-afternoon snack
Fresh vegetable juice or hot or iced herbal tea
10 raw nuts: almonds, walnuts, or pecans

Dinner
Spicy Chicken Salad (p. 194)
Blue Cornmeal Muffin (p. 223)

DAY 5

Make this a vegetarian day.

Breakfast
Fresh vegetable juice
Fluffy Cheese Omelet (p. 182)
Sliced fresh tomatoes with drizzle of balsamic vinegar and
  chopped herbs

Mid-morning snack
1 Granny Smith or pippin apple
Hot or iced herbal tea with lemon

Lunch

Hummus (p. 204) and vegetable sticks

Spinach salad with Lemon–Olive Oil Dressing (p. 201) or dressing of choice

Hearty Split Pea Soup (p. 188)

Mid-afternoon snack

6 raw almonds

Hot or iced herbal tea

Dinner

Red Lentil–Rice Patties with Coconut-Cilantro Sauce (p. 209)

Spring Greens, Red Onion, and Orange Salad with Curry-
Orange Dressing (p. 197)

Dessert

Fresh Strawberries with Coconut Sauce (p. 225)

DAY 6

Breakfast

Vegetable juice

Scrambled eggs

Sliced fresh tomatoes with chopped fresh herbs

Herbal tea with lemon

Mid-morning snack

1 slice of turkey

3 radishes and 4 cucumber slices

Lunch
Grilled or smoked salmon over bed of greens with choice of
dressing
Gazpacho (p. 192)

Mid-afternoon snack
Hot or iced herbal tea
6 raw almonds

Dinner
Caesar Salad (p. 198)
Baked chicken
Dressed-up Broccoli (p. 219)

DAY 7

Breakfast
Fresh vegetable juice
Oatmeal (not instant), amaranth, or quinoa
Almond or rice milk
Fresh berries (blueberries, blackberries, raspberries, or straw-
berries)
Healthy low-carb sweetener (optional)
Herbal tea with lemon

Mid-morning snack
4 celery sticks stuffed with almond butter
Hot or iced herbal tea with lemon

Lunch
Basic Garden Salad (p. 193) with choice of dressing
One cup garden vegetable soup

Mid-afternoon snack
Iced herbal tea with lemon
6 raw pecans

Dinner
Lemon-Artichoke Salad (p. 199)
Baked Flounder (p. 211)
Grilled zucchini and yellow summer squash
Herbal tea with lemon

DAY 8

Make this a vegetarian day.

Breakfast
Green or herbal tea with lemon
Fresh vegetable juice
1–2 soft-boiled eggs
1 slice whole multigrain or sprouted-grain bread spread with
   butter, coconut oil, or almond butter

Mid-morning snack
Iced or hot herbal tea
1 piece low-sugar fruit

Lunch
Lima Bean Soup (p. 189)
Veggie sticks
Savory Rosemary-Onion Muffin (p. 224)

Mid-afternoon snack
Sparkling mineral water with a slice of lemon or lime
6 raw or toasted almonds

Dinner
Basic Garden Salad (p. 193) with choice of dressing
Millet-Walnut Stuffed Peppers (p. 212)
Steamed green beans with sliced almonds

DAY 9

Breakfast
Green or herbal tea with lemon
Scrambled eggs
1 or 2 slices turkey bacon

Mid-morning snack
6–8 ounces vegetable juice, preferably made fresh
6 raw or toasted almonds

Lunch
Red Lentil–Spinach Soup (p. 190)
Spinach salad with choice of dressing
Savory Onion-Rosemary Muffin (p. 224)

Mid-afternoon snack
Sparkling mineral water with a slice of lemon
Vegetable sticks

Dinner
Basic Garden Salad (p. 193) with Asian Dressing (p. 203)
Grilled Salmon (p. 213)
Grilled vegetable medley

DAY 10

Breakfast
Green or herbal tea with lemon
Strawberry-Coconut Smoothie (p. 180)

Mid-morning snack
Fresh vegetable juice

Lunch
Caesar Salad (p. 198) with Grilled Salmon (p. 213) left over from
    the day before
Blue Cornmeal Muffin (p. 223)

Mid-afternoon snack
Sparkling mineral water with a slice of lemon
6 pecans

Dinner
Basic Garden Salad (p. 193) with dressing of choice
Fish Tacos (p. 214)

DAY 11

Breakfast
Green or herbal tea with lemon
Fresh vegetable juice
Basic scrambled eggs
2 slices turkey bacon

Mid-morning snack
Herbal tea with lemon
6 Brazil nuts

Lunch
Tomato stuffed with tuna salad
2 dehydrated seed crackers or rye crisps

Mid-afternoon snack
Sparkling mineral water with a slice of lemon
1 celery rib stuffed with soft goat cheese, cut into six pieces

Dinner
Basic Garden Salad (p. 193) with your favorite vinaigrette
Spicy and Crispy Broiled Halibut (p. 215)
Kale with Garlic and Red Pepper (p. 220)

DAY 12

Breakfast
Green or herbal tea with lemon
Fresh vegetable juice
Mediterranean Frittata (p. 183)

Mid-morning snack
Fresh vegetable juice
6 raw almonds

Lunch
Tuscan Sun White Bean Soup (p. 191)
Tomato-mozzarella salad with fresh basil and a drizzle of balsamic
    vinegar and extra-virgin olive oil

Mid-afternoon snack
Sparkling mineral water with a slice of lemon or lime
2 thin slices turkey breast

Dinner
Basic Garden Salad (p. 193) with choice of dressing
Grilled Pepper-Crusted Chicken (p. 216)
Steamed green beans

DAY 13

Breakfast
Green or herbal tea with lemon
Fresh vegetable juice of choice

1 poached egg
1 slice multigrain bread, toasted
2 strips turkey bacon

Mid-morning snack
Herbal or green tea with lemon
6 to 10 pecans

Lunch
Grilled-chicken Caesar salad (you can use leftover chicken from
    the day before)

Mid-afternoon snack
Sparkling mineral water with a slice of lemon
Veggie sticks with Hummus (p. 204)

Dinner
Sliced tomatoes sprinkled with Italian herbs of choice and a driz-
    zle of extra-virgin olive oil
Creamed Turkey with Mushrooms (p. 217)
Wild and brown rice
Steamed asparagus and globe artichokes

DAY 14

Breakfast
Green or herbal tea with lemon
Fresh vegetable juice
Eggs Benedict Florentine (p. 184)

Mid-morning snack
Green or herbal tea with lemon
6 macadamia nuts

Lunch
Smoked salmon on a bed of greens with your choice of dressing

Mid-afternoon snack
Sparkling mineral water with lemon
3 radishes and 4 olives

Dinner
Multigrain Florentine Salad (p. 200)
Mediterranean Rice Pilaf (p. 221)

Dessert
Fresh Strawberry Pie with Coconut Crust (p. 226)

THE NEXT STEP

Now that you've finished Step 2, and your body has had a chance to gently begin the detoxification process, you are ready for Step 3. With the cleansing programs, you should see some amazing results in how you feel, look, and think. As you rid your body of toxins, waste, and old stored water, you should feel lighter, healthier, and younger. As you de-junk your body and recharge your life, you'll be giving your body a break and your life an instant lift! You're about to follow a cleansing plan that can reclaim a measure of youth you may have thought was gone forever. Get ready to feel brand-spanking-new!

Step 3: The Cleansing Boost Programs

Now that you've finished Step 2, the14-Day Wrinkle Cleanse Diet, and you have gently detoxified your body for two weeks, it's time to add a boost to your Wrinkle Cleanse program. Step 3, the cleansing boost programs, will give you an opportunity to experience deeper cleansing in the organs of your body, like the kind of spring cleaning you might give your home. The cleansing boost programs are designed to clean out your intestinal tract, liver, gallbladder, kidneys, and at the same time get rid of old stored water and purify the blood. These programs can totally transform your face and your health. Like many other people, you may lose wrinkles, unwanted weight, and a host of health problems, too.

As you've already learned, a toxic body is one of the major contributors to the aging process and an underlying reason for wrinkles, sagging skin, and many other aspects of aging, including disease. The body does naturally detox, but the body's defenses may not be enough today, because of all the environmental pollutants and tobacco smoke we're exposed to and all the "pigging out" and alcohol consumption that we indulge in.

Cleansing (also known as detoxification) of the body is an important step in slowing and reversing aging. You can pour bushels of nutrients into your body, but if it's toxic, congested, and the cells are not functioning well at taking in nutrients and expelling waste, all those super nutrients will not do you a great deal of good. It's a bit like continuing to wax a floor over and over again, without ever stripping it. Dirt and grime can build up and all the new wax applied over and over will never produce a sparkling clean floor until you strip off all the old stuff. When you do, that first coat of wax makes a big difference in how the floor shines.

There are a variety of cleanses to choose from in this chapter, each one designed to provide you with some extra help in ridding the target organ of toxins and your face of lines and wrinkles. Without these special cleanses, the organs of elimination may never get completely cleansed and therefore may never operate at peak performance. Just how does "really cleansed" relate to your face? You might say it could be likened to cleaning your windows on the inside as well as the outside or taking a scrub brush to the corners of your shower. When you're done, everything looks brand-spanking new again.

The colon, liver, gallbladder, and kidneys are among our hardest-working organs, yet we forget about them because we can't see them. We can really help them by giving them a rest and a "spring cleaning" every year. Detoxification is the method of "spring cleaning" that helps us eliminate wastes and toxins from the body that may have been stored up for a long time.

Each of the cleanses in this program is designed to work with the 14-Day Wrinkle Cleanse Diet. You will continue with this diet—it represents your new antiwrinkle lifestyle—while adding the cleansing boost programs. Your diet will consist of the life-giving foods you have been eating for two weeks, and you will add the special dietary elements outlined in each of the cleansing boost programs. As you work your way through the programs, you will discover that the benefits are enormous.

You'll begin with the colon cleanse, which is designed to help strip away waste that has accumulated on the intestinal wall and that hinders good nutrient absorption and waste elimination. If you think that stuff stuck to the intestinal wall sounds rather strange, I did too, until I tried my first colon cleanse. It was 1996 and my face looked puffy and my skin was sagging. I was looking older and less vibrant than today. About a week into the colon cleanse, there before my eyes were the results of the cleansing process, just as Dr. Richard Anderson (*Cleanse and Purify Thyself*) and Dr. Bernard Jensen (*Tissue Cleansing Through Bowel Management*) had described in their books. The colon cleanse was stripping material off my intestinal walls that had obviously been around a long time. My face started showing the positive results of cleansing—within a couple of weeks the puffiness was nearly gone and my skin had tightened some and looked more vibrant.

I often look at the faces of rather young women and occasionally notice brown discoloration around the lips, especially above the upper lip. (Brown discoloration above the lip and a grayish or less-than-vibrant complexion can be signs of colon toxicity.) As the colon is cleansed, the skin should become clearer and more vibrant and any brown discoloration should disappear. A medical doctor who specialized in nutrition advised me years ago that a brown tan line above the upper lip could be a sign of a colon polyp (a tumorous growth that can be benign or malignant). I had such a line above my upper lip at the time. That line went away after a five-day vegetable juice fast cleanse along with a polyp (turns out I did have one).

Once the colon is cleansed, you're ready for the liver cleanse and then the gallbladder cleanse. The gallbladder is a supporting organ to the liver and congestion in this organ can hinder the liver's important work, so it's essential to cleanse them both. It is also important that the intestinal tract is cleansed so that when toxins are released from the liver and the gallbladder, they can easily make their way out of the body. The liver and gallbladder cleanses incorporate dietary ingredients that help to purge these vital organs of congestion, waste matter, and toxins. In Chinese medicine, brown spots (from freckles to age spots) and red spots on the skin are considered signs that the liver and gallbladder are in need of rest and cleansing. As these organs are detoxified, brown spots may lessen or disappear (hardened red spots are harder to get rid of; it usually takes a dermatological procedure known as hyfrecation— a professional process that burns them off).

When I undertook the liver and gallbladder cleanses for the first time, I was amazed to see what was released from my body and encouraged by how my digestion improved. And weight (about five pounds) just melted off! Weight loss is not a big deal when the liver is cleansed. The liver is the fat burner of the body, and when it's detoxified, fat burning accelerates and weight loss becomes easier. (Many people can't lose weight because of a poorly functioning, congested liver. Often, those who say they eat almost nothing and still don't lose weight desperately need a liver cleanse.)

The kidney cleanse is the fourth cleanse in the program. The kidneys can get very taxed, just like the other organs of elimination, with all the chemicals, caffeine, medications, alcohol, and junk food that Westerners typically ingest. In Chinese medicine, dark circles around the eyes correspond to overburdened kidneys. As the kidneys are cleansed, dark circles should gradually disappear, elimination should improve, and edema and facial puffiness should lessen.

Although I can point to a host of specific benefits of each cleanse, all cleanses work together to roll back the years and supercharge your 14-Day Wrinkle Cleanse. I recommend that you work your way through the cleansing boost programs in the order that they are presented, unless you are otherwise advised by your health-care professional, in order to experience the best results.

Cleanse Boosters

As you cleanse your body, you can further assist the process with a variety of body-pampering actions. Here are some suggestions to help you feel fabulous as you clean your "inner house."

- Massage
- Facial or at-home facial steam bath with rosemary, lavender, or peppermint
- Face pack: Mix together two tablespoons each of plain yogurt, fine (not instant) oatmeal, and cleansing herbs such as thyme leaves, chamomile, elder flowers, violet, yarrow, or fennel leaves. Apply to face, lie down for ten minutes, and then rinse with cool water.
- Sauna, especially a far-infrared sauna, and steam helps you sweat away toxins
- Essential oil rub: Rub peppermint, rosemary, or mandarin oil in a circular motion around your abdomen to improve digestion and elimination of toxins
- Mud bath: White clay boosts circulation and lymphatic flow
- Body brushing removes dead skin cells and other debris
- A sea salt and soda bath helps detox. Add one cup of each to your bathwater and soak for thirty minutes to draw out the toxins.
- A salt glow rub sloughs off dead skin cells. Massage a paste made of sea salt and water into your skin. Rub in a circular

motion, starting with your feet and working up to your arms; rinse in the shower. (Avoid delicate skin areas such as around your eyes.)

- Rejuvenate with a lemon oil bath
- Take a twenty-minute health-shop–bought seaweed bath to purge toxins
- Rest and relax more
- Take a nap
- Get an extra hour of sleep
- Spend some time each day outside in the fresh air
- Meditate or pray
- Clean out a closet or drawer that's messy; you'll feel much better looking at the neat space

THE COLON CLEANSE PROGRAM

Although I refer to it as the colon cleanse, this program is a complete intestinal cleanse. The small and large intestines comprise about twenty-six feet of twists and folds within the body. The small intestine is made up of three segments: duodenum, jejunum, and ileum. The large intestine, also known as the colon, is also made up of three segments: ascending, transverse, and descending. The small intestine is where most of the minerals, vitamins, carbohydrates, proteins, fat, cholesterol, and bile salts are absorbed. Some nutrients and water are also absorbed in the colon and this is where the stool is formed. (About two-thirds of the stool is water, undigested fiber, and food products, and about one-third is living and dead bacteria.)

Because the formation and build-up of intestinal toxins can undermine our appearance as well as our health, it is imperative to cleanse the entire intestinal tract. Intestinal problems start with foods such as highly refined, low-fiber foods and many of the substances they contain such as preservatives, pesticides, dyes, sugars, and fillers. We may eat too many mucus-forming foods such as dairy products, refined flour products, and sweets, or ingest irritating substances such as alcohol, caffeine, and preservatives that cause excessive mucous secretions. Prescription drugs can cause irritation and congestion. We may not drink enough water or get enough exercise. And we may have endocrine disorders such as low thyroid, elevated calcium levels, or pituitary disorders. All these factors contribute to a sluggish colon, which means slow transit time, known as constipation.

The intestines can store a large amount of waste in the form of partially digested, putrefying matter. When we don't eliminate this waste at least once but preferably two or three times a day, toxins from the feces are absorbed back into the bloodstream. These toxins include free radicals, which cause oxidative stress and result in damaged cells. This leads to damaging effects on the skin as well as the entire body, as discussed in Chapter 1.

As waste sits in the colon, substances such as old fecal matter and mucus can become lodged or stuck to the lining of the intestinal tract. In his book *Cleanse and Purify Thyself,* Richard Anderson, ND, calls this material *mucoid plaque.* Once mucoid plaque is created, it is not routinely eliminated. Rather, it lodges in the numerous folds and crevices of the intestinal tract and can remain there for years. Old feces can adhere to the plaque and may not be removed during normal elimination. (This can be a contributor to diverticulosis.) Plaque slows down bowel action, thus slowing waste elimination, and causing more toxins to be reabsorbed into the system. This contributes to more free radicals and inflammation and inhibits nutrient absorption. And the plaque can harbor pathogens such as bacteria and parasites and block the release of lymph and mucus.

The colon cleanse will not only improve digestion and elimination, it will help to slow down aging. People who have incorporated the colon cleansing process into their lifestyle, along with a whole foods, high-antioxidant diet, often notice a softening or disappearance of wrinkles, a tightening of their skin, and a brighter, more glowing complexion.

Complete colon cleansing can take up to six weeks, especially if you've never cleansed your intestinal tract before, and it's worth it. The best approach is to thoroughly cleanse the intestines, but after a week or two, you can add the liver cleanse to the colon cleanse, then the gall-bladder cleanse, and finally the kidney cleanse. The goal is to have a week or two to clear the colon of a lot of waste before your liver starts releasing toxins, so that they will have a clearer channel and be expelled efficiently.

For the entire process of cleansing, you should follow the 14-Day Wrinkle Cleanse Diet and include plenty of raw foods such as vegetables, vegetable juices, fresh fruit, sprouts, salad greens, nuts, and seeds with each meal. For the duration of the colon cleanse, you will supplement your diet with fiber shakes and colon-cleanse herbal supplements. If you wish to go on a stricter phase of colon cleansing, you can substitute an additional fiber shake for one meal, either lunch or dinner. Make sure to get plenty of water (a minimum of sixty-four ounces per day) plus one to two glasses of fresh vegetable juice. Also, be sure to get plenty of rest; your body is working hard to get rid of junk, and this is the time to assist it.

I recommend you start each day with a freshly made glass of vegetable juice and as a mid-morning or afternoon snack, prepare a freshly made green juice (or take one to work in a thermos) or, if that is not possible, powdered greens can be mixed in water or with V-8 juice. Mineral supplements, extra vitamin C, and a colon flush are optional elements of the colon cleanse program, but they can be valuable boosts to your detoxification.

THE COLON CLEANSE MENU

Though at first glance the colon cleanse can look like it would be impossible to carry out while working outside the home, it is actually not that hard. Look closely at the menu for the morning and afternoon program and you'll see that most of the entries are water. The fiber shakes could easily be made at work in a jar or plastic container while on break. Herbal tea is easy to carry with you. If you want fresh juice, you can make it at home and take it to work in a thermos or you can go out for it. Juice stands are becoming more popular in malls and shopping centers. Or you can take powdered greens and mix with V-8 juice. Herbal supplements are easy to pack along as well. And even if you always eat lunch out, almost every restaurant has main course salads and other healthy fare to choose from. This program can work, even with a busy work schedule. It just means taking a couple of breaks during the day and planning ahead for what you will take to work.

Breakfast
7: 00 a.m.: Fiber shake (see p. 136)

7:15 a.m.: Herbal tea with lemon or hot water with lemon

7:30 a.m.: Freshly made vegetable juice

Breakfast: Choose from the breakfast recipes in Chapter 8 and add some raw food such as sliced tomatoes, avocado, or fresh berries

Recommended: Additional minerals (either liquid minerals or capsules)

Morning program

9:00 a.m.: 8 ounces of water

9:30 a.m.: Herbs: intestinal cleansing herbal supplements

10:00 a.m.: 8 ounces water or freshly made vegetable juice

10:30 a.m.: Fiber shake

11:00 a.m.: 8 ounces water

11:30 a.m.: 8 ounces water

Lunch

Noon: Choose from the lunch recipes in Chapter 8 and add some raw food

Afternoon program

1: 30 p.m.: Herbs: cleansing herbal supplements (see p. 137) (depending on the brand, supplements may not be called for at this time)

2:00 p.m.: 8 ounces water or sparkling water with lemon

2:30 p.m.: 8 ounces water or sparkling water with lemon

3:00 p.m.: Fiber shake

3:30 p.m.: 8 ounces water or sparkling water with lemon

4:00 p.m.: 8 ounces water or sparkling water with lemon

4:30 p.m.: Herbs: cleansing herbal supplements (depending on the brand, supplements may not be called for at this time)

5:00 p.m.: 8 ounces water or sparkling water with lemon

Dinner

5:30–6:00 p.m.: Choose from the dinner recipes in Chapter 8 and add some raw food such as a green salad

8:00 p.m.: Herbal tea such as peppermint or chamomile

FIBER SHAKE

You'll need three ingredients to make your fiber shakes:

- Bentonite clay acts like a magnet or sponge that absorbs material such as toxins, bacteria, and parasites from the intestinal tract. It should be used with fiber. As it pulls the plaque from the intestinal wall, the matter will adhere to the fiber and be swept away. Available in powder or liquid (I recommend liquid as better).
- Psyllium or ground flax fiber swells when mixed with liquid and acts like a broom in the intestinal tract, sweeping it clean of loosened substances.
- Cranberry juice is cleansing for the kidneys and black cherry juice is good for the colon and adds flavor to the shake. (Both can be found in unsweetened concentrates at most health food stores.) I recommend one teaspoon of either.
- All of these items are readily available at health food stores.

RECIPE FOR COLON CLEANSE

Fiber Shake

1 scoop fiber (according to directions)
1 tablespoon liquid bentonite clay (or according to directions)
6 to 8 ounces water
1 teaspoon unsweetened pure cranberry juice extract or black cherry extract for flavor (optional)

Mix fiber and bentonite clay with water in a jar or plastic container. Add cranberry juice extract or black cherry juice extract, as desired, to the mixture and shake vigorously.

Makes 1 shake

CLEANSING HERBS

A variety of herbal programs are available that you can use for colon cleansing. My favorites are by Arise & Shine (psyllium, bentonite, herbal nutrition, and chomper) and Advanced Naturals (Fiber Max and Cleanse Max I and II; see Resources p. 250). These herbs help to break up intestinal plaque, remove waste, and give nutritional support to the intestines. Without cleansing herbs, the colon cleanse is not nearly as effective.

PROBIOTICS

Probiotics are the friendly bacteria that live inside each of us in vast numbers; without sufficient numbers of them we will not experience good health. They perform many important functions within the body and different bacteria have unique roles. For example, some friendly bacteria produce antibacterial substances that kill or deactivate unfriendly, disease-causing bacteria, viruses, and yeasts. And they improve the efficiency of the digestive tract. If they are weakened, such as by taking antibiotics or other medications, bowel function is poor. Types of friendly bacteria include: lactobacillus acidophilus, lactobacillus bulgaricus, bifidobacterium bifidum, and bifidobacterium longum.

Cleansing the intestinal tract will remove both good and bad bacteria. Therefore, following an intestinal cleanse, it is important to finish with probiotics to replenish the good bacteria. After the intestinal tract is cleansed is the best time for good bacteria to become well established. If you eat plenty of raw vegetables and fruit in addition to taking probiotics, you will be on your way to improved intestinal health and to looking and feeling younger. There are a variety of probiotics available. You should take them according to the directions and finish the bottle.

Water

It is very important to get at least eight to ten 8-ounce glasses of water each day, not only to hydrate your body, which helps prevent wrinkles, but also to flush out toxins while you cleanse. You may need more than 64 ounces of water per day, as this amount is recommended for a person weighing around 120 pounds. If you weigh more, drink a minimum of ten glasses of water a day. Also, if you live at a high altitude or in a dry climate you'll need at least ten glasses of water daily.

Minerals

Liquid minerals are an optional part of the colon cleanse program, but I recommend them for detoxification support as well as improved health. Be aware that as you pull toxins out of the intestinal tract, minerals may be pulled out with them and it's important to replace them. In terms of cleansing, minerals assist metabolic enzymes in their role of detoxifying and rebuilding cells. People supplementing with minerals have reported a variety of visible improvements such as gray hair returning to its former color and rashes disappearing.

The minerals recommended in Resources, page 251, are in a state small enough to be easily utilized by the body.

COLON FLUSH (COLONIC OR ENEMA)

Colon hydrotherapy, which is popularly known as a *colonic,* entails flushing the colon with water, usually by a professional colonic therapist. Colon hydrotherapy is a safe, effective method of removing waste from the large intestine without the use of drugs. Intestinal waste is softened and loosened by introducing pure, filtered, and temperature-regulated water into the colon, which results in the evacuation of waste. A colonic or two per week during the four to six weeks of colon cleansing is particularly helpful to remove excess waste. It can also be helpful in facilitating weight loss.

When you are detoxifying, more toxins can build up in the intestinal tract than your body can eliminate quickly and efficiently, and that can lead to headaches, flu-type symptoms, and a host of other reactions known as the Herxheimer Reaction. Flushing the colon offers quick relief from such symptoms, and it also offers protection from toxins being reabsorbed back into the system.

If you're thinking, No way would I consider this, it might be of interest to know that some of the most glamorous people we watch in the media have taken advantage of this health practice. Princess Diana was said to have been an avid fan of colonics. And it's rumored that numerous Hollywood stars get colonics. The reason partakers range from royalty to Hollywood to people like us is that colonics help to reduce bloating and gas, flatten protruding tummies, facilitate weight loss, improve colon health, clear the whites of the eyes, add luminescence to the skin, and assist people in looking younger. Everyone benefits from flushing the colon.

While it might be disconcerting to the very shy, most practitioners will immediately make you feel relaxed, at ease, and safe. Just make sure the center you choose is clean and uses disposable hoses and tubes.

If you are unable to find a colon therapist in your area, the next best thing is an enema, which you can administer yourself. Look in your local drugstore for an enema bag if you don't have one, and follow the directions.

The Herxheimer Reaction

The detoxification phenomenon is often referred to as a "healing crisis" or the Herxheimer Reaction. When toxins are released faster than the body can process, we can experience symptoms such as headaches, stomachaches, diarrhea, increased thirst, loss of appetite, fatigue, or irritability. Should you experience any of these symptoms, drink plenty of water and make sure the colon is flushed, which should ease the symptoms. Detoxification reactions actually are a good sign that you're doing all the right things and your body is getting rid of toxic material that contributes to aging and disease.

THE LIVER CLEANSE PROGRAM

Though the liver has many roles such as carbohydrate, protein, and fat metabolism; storage of vitamins and minerals; and production of bile, its primary work is to detoxify the body. While the skin is the largest organ of the body, the liver is the largest internal organ. Filtering and purifying the blood; removing drugs, toxins, and poisons; and keeping body fluids clean are vital roles of the liver. Making sure all the fluids are clean is key to your antiaging program, because these fluids are the internal "fountain of youth," as discussed in Chapter 1. When they are cleansed, our cells are able to better eliminate waste and take in nutrients.

The liver has to deal with more toxic materials today than at any time in history. Substances such as chemical water treatments, pesticides, chemical fertilizers, food additives, and industrial pollution bombard us daily. Add to that overconsumption of alcohol, caffeine, preservatives, sugar and sweets, damaged fats, refined and processed foods, and we have a perfect setup for a distressed liver. Constant abuse of the liver contributes to aging and disease. Therefore, cleansing the liver so that it can function well is a key factor in your wrinkle cleanse program. And if you have had your gallbladder removed, you need periodic liver cleansing even more.

The Liver, Thyroid, Gallstones, and Antiaging

Philip G. Young, MD, author of *Thyroid: Guardian of Health,* says that the liver processes cholesterol, which is turned into bile, and that this is important in the digestion of fats. This process becomes sluggish in hypothyroid individuals. Cholesterol stones then form in the gallbladder. (Gallbladder attack is frequent in hypothyroidism.) When this happens, the liver tends to get clogged with excessive cholesterol and may not function properly unless it is cleansed.

When the thyroid is undernourished and not functioning well, we can experience symptoms such as dry skin, difficulty losing weight, sleep disturbances, headaches, fatigue, depression, and recurrent infections— all factors that can cause us to look older. Thyroid tests are not designed to detect an undernourished and slightly low functioning thyroid. (Take the Thyroid Quiz, p. 240, if you suspect you may have an underactive thyroid.) A healthy liver is one of the keys to a well-functioning thyroid gland; T4 is converted to T3 (thyroid hormones) primarily in the liver. As you cleanse and support your liver, you may notice your thyroid function improving, and consequently, so will your sleep, dry skin, resistance to infections, weight loss, and a host of other annoying symptoms. And, lo and behold—you're looking younger!

Sandra Cabot, MD, author of *The Liver Cleansing Diet,* shares testimonies in her book of two ladies from Australia (Cabot's country of medical practice) who detoxed their livers and reaped a bundle of rewards. Ms. H got rid of a host of aches and pains and discovered that her "tired looking skin again has a glow about it" that even her friends comment on. And Ms. J reported that after eleven weeks on the liver cleansing diet, her acne rosacea was gone and she had lost forty-eight pounds.

It is best to embark on the liver cleanse following at least one to two weeks on the colon cleanse, so that when the liver starts releasing toxins, the body will be able to move them through the intestinal tract quickly. The liver cleanse week is easy to follow and it offers huge rewards not only for your face, but also for your health. During this week you will continue with the 14-Day Wrinkle Cleanse Diet, and will be adding raw veggies or fresh vegetable juices with each meal, plus a beet salad, carrot salad, mineral-rich vegetable broth, and liver cleanse herbs and supplements, as desired, each day.

THE LIVER CLEANSE MENU

Breakfast

7:00 a.m. or upon rising: Drink 1 cup hot water with the juice of
¼ lemon and a dash of cayenne pepper

7:15 a.m.: Liver Cleanse Cocktail (p. 146)

7:30 a.m.: Choose from the breakfast entrées in Chapter 8 and
include some raw food such as sliced tomatoes, avocado, or
fresh berries

Supplement: 1 or 2 capsules of the herb milk thistle or other liver-
cleansing herbal supplements (pp. 149–50)

Morning program

9:00 a.m.: 1 to 2 teaspoons Beet Salad (p. 147)

9:30 a.m.: 8 ounces of water

10:00 a.m.: Herbal tea with lemon

10:30 a.m.: 8 ounces of water

11:00 a.m.: 1 to 2 teaspoons Beet Salad (p. 147)

11:30 a.m.: 8 ounces of water

Lunch

12:00 noon: Choose from the lunch entrées in Chapter 8 and add
some raw food such as a green salad, veggie sticks, vegetable
juice, gazpacho, or sliced tomatoes

Supplement: 1 to 2 capsules of the herb milk thistle or other liver-
cleansing herbal supplements (pp. 149–50)

Afternoon program

1:30 p.m.: 1 to 2 teaspoons Beet Salad (p. 147)

2:00 p.m.: 8 ounces of water

2:30 p.m.: 10 ounces Green Drink (p. 147)

3:00 p.m.: 8 ounces of water

3:30 p.m.: 1 to 2 teaspoons Beet Salad (p. 147)

4:00 p.m.: 8 ounces of water

4:30 p.m.: Herbal tea with lemon

5:30 p.m.: 1 to 2 teaspoons Beet Salad (p. 147)

Dinner

6:00 p.m.: Carrot Salad (p. 148)

One cup Mineral-Rich Vegetable Broth (p. 148)

Main course salad or dinner entrée of choice from Chapter 8 with some raw food

Supplement: 1 to 2 capsules milk thistle or other liver-cleansing herbal supplements (pp. 149–50)

7:15 p.m.: 1 to 2 teaspoons Beet Salad (p. 147)

8:30 p.m.: Chamomile or peppermint herbal tea

Note: *Avoid eating after 7:30 p.m., to give your liver a chance to do its work of cleansing.*

The Liver Cleanse Foods and Recipes

Eat More Liver-Friendly Foods

During this week, you can benefit by eating more foods that have been shown to support the liver. You may never have eaten some of the foods listed here, or even noticed them at the market. Now is a perfect time to expand your dietary horizons and try a few new foods.

Artichokes	Kale
Beans	Kohlrabi
Beets	Mustard greens
Broccoli	Okra
Brussels sprouts	Onion
Cabbage	Parsley
Carrots	Peas
Cauliflower	Parsnips
Celery	Pumpkin
Chives	Sweet potatoes
Cucumber	Squash
Eggplant	Yams
Garlic	

Hot Water with Lemon and Cayenne Pepper

Lemon and cayenne pepper in hot water is a traditional morning tonic used for liver cleansing to help stimulate the liver and gallbladder. Lemon juice has long been used for liver and gallbladder cleansing. Capsicum (cayenne pepper) is a catalyst in blood purification that helps stimulate the organs of elimination to greater activity. It also acts as a diaphoretic, which means it stimulates excretion of wastes in sweat. (You may also benefit by taking a cayenne pepper capsule each day.) Mix the juice of ¼ lemon with 1 cup hot water and a dash of cayenne.

Liver Cleanse Cocktail

- 1 handful fresh parsley
- 4 medium carrots, scrubbed well, green tops removed, ends trimmed
- 1 small or ½ medium beet with stems and leaves, scrubbed well
- 1 cucumber (peeled, if not organic)
- 2 stalks celery with leaves, washed, ends trimmed
- ½ lemon, peeled
- 2-inch piece ginger root, peeled

Bunch up the parsley and push it through the juicer feed tube with the carrots, beet, cucumber, celery, lemon, and ginger. Stir the juice and pour into a glass. Drink as soon as possible to maximize the nutritional value or store in the refrigerator, covered, or take with you in a thermos.

Makes 1 to 2 servings

Nutritional analysis: 371 calories (7% from fat) • 3g fat • 12g protein • 84g carbohydrate • >2g dietary fiber • 0mg cholesterol • 300mg sodium

Beet Salad

~~~~~

2 tablespoons extra-virgin olive oil
Juice of ½ lemon, preferably organic
1 cup raw beets, finely grated or chopped, preferably organic

Whisk the olive oil and lemon juice together and add the grated beets. Eat one to two teaspoons of this salad every two hours during an eight-hour period for seven days.

Makes 1 cup

Nutritional analysis (per 1 cup serving): 330 calories (75% from fat) • 28g fat • 3g protein • 5g fiber • 18g carbohydrate • 0mg cholesterol • 132mg sodium • 190mcg folic acid • 590mg potassium • 40mg magnesium

Green Drink

~~~~~

Juice as many greens as you like. Start with a base of cucumber, celery, and lemon. To that you can add parsley, kale, spinach, or sprouts. You can also add fresh mint or ginger root to improve the flavor. Or, if you don't have a juicer, use the powdered greens available at most health food stores. You can add some lemon juice to improve the flavor. Fresh vegetable juices are also available at supermarkets and health food stores.

Carrot Salad

~~~~~~

1 cup finely shredded carrots, or carrot pulp left over from juicing
1 tablespoon extra-virgin olive oil
1 tablespoon fresh lemon juice
1 dash cinnamon

Place shredded carrots in a bowl. (The carrots should be a mushy consistency; use a food processor or fine grater, or use the carrot pulp.) In another bowl, whisk together olive oil, lemon juice, and cinnamon to make dressing (you may add more dressing, but not less). Pour the dressing over the carrots and mix well.

Makes 1 cup

Nutritional analysis (per 1 cup serving): 180 calories (69% from fat) • 14g fat • 1g protein • 3.5g fiber • 12g carbohydrate • 0mg cholesterol • 38mg sodium • 377mg potassium

Mineral-Rich Vegetable Broth

This vegetable broth recipe provides important nutrients, especially minerals, your body needs during the cleansing process. Eat one to two cups of the broth daily.

2 to 3 cups chopped fresh string beans (frozen is acceptable when fresh is not available)
2 to 3 cups chopped zucchini
2 to 3 stalks celery

1 to 3 tablespoons chopped parsley
1 tablespoon chopped garlic
Fresh ginger root, cayenne, or herbs to taste

Steam the string beans, zucchini, and celery over purified water until soft, but still green and not mushy. Place the cooked vegetables, plus the raw parsley and garlic, in a blender and purée until smooth. Add a bit of the steaming water, as needed, but keep the broth fairly thick. Season to taste with minced ginger, cayenne, or herbs of your choice.

Makes about 6 cups

Nutritional analysis (per 1 cup serving): 53 calories (5% from fat) • 0.3g fat • 2.5g protein • 4.5g fiber • 12g carbohydrate • 0mg cholesterol • 284mg sodium • 578mg potassium • 46mg magnesium • 63mg calcium

MILK THISTLE (SILYMARIN)

Take one to two capsules (recommended dosage is 70 to 210 mg) of the herb milk thistle three times per day with a meal. Milk thistle contains some of the most potent liver-cleansing compounds known. Silymarin, the most active ingredient in milk thistle, enhances liver function. It also has excellent antioxidant properties that help prevent damage to the liver.

Other Beneficial Liver Cleanse Supplements (Optional)

Lipotropic Formula. Nutritional supplements known as lipotropic formulas containing choline, betaine, and/or methionine and cysteine are designed to promote the flow of fat and bile to and from the liver. They are formulated to improve liver function and enhance detoxification. For the best effect, you will need to get a daily dose of 1,000 mg choline and 1,000 mg of either methionine or cysteine.

Solvent Removal Support. There are specific amino acids and other nutrients that are specific to solvent detoxification in the liver: glycine, glutamine, taurine (150 mg each), N-acetyl-L-cysteine (50 mg), and alpha lipoic acid (50 mg).

Formaldehyde Removal Support. Outgassing from new carpet and furniture, *Candida albicans,* and alcohol metabolism contain aldehydes, formaldehyde being one of the most common of the aldehydes. Thiamine (25 mg), pyridoxine (50 mg), selenium (50 mg), and pantethine (100 mg) can be very helpful in assisting in the detoxification of these compounds.

Liver Cleansing Thoughts

Chinese medicine says that anger results in stoppage of bile flow, or liver stagnation, resulting in fermentation and heat, which causes "fire to rise." This leads to agitation, poor sleep, and headaches. If you feel agitated or somewhat "hyped-up," it could be because your liver is full of toxins and in need of a cleanse. As you cleanse the toxins, cleanse your emotions, too. Forgiveness and "letting go" of negative thoughts are antidotes to anger, and joy produces an increase in bile flow.

THE GALLBLADDER CLEANSE

The gallbladder is a supporting organ of elimination. Its function is to store and concentrate bile. One of the body's primary methods of eliminating toxins is via the bile, a yellowish-green fluid produced in the liver and stored in the gallbladder. It passes through ducts to the small intestine, where it plays an essential role in emulsifying fats. Because good-quality bile is important for elimination of toxins, it is essential that we care for the gallbladder and support its function. If your gallbladder has been removed, it is even more important to care for your liver.

Our typical Western diet, which is rich in foods that contribute to gallstones and gallbladder congestion, does not support good gallbladder function. To maintain a healthy gallbladder, the gallbladder cleanse is a key part of the Wrinkle Cleanse program. Once you have completed the gallbladder cleanse, you may notice that digestion, particularly digestion of fats, and weight management improve. Former problems such as bloating, gas, and belching may be gone, and you'll be one step further along to a younger-looking you.

The gallbladder cleanse is designed to soften stones and increase bile solubility. Continue with the Wrinkle Cleanse Diet and make sure you eat only small amounts of lean protein (about a 4-ounce serving; no more than twice a day) during this week, reduce your animal fat intake significantly, and increase your intake of raw food—fresh vegetables, vegetable juice, low-sugar fruit, sprouts, and salad greens, with good fats, particularly the omega-3 fatty acids, and whole grains and legumes. During this cleansing week, you will be adding vegetable juice cleansing cocktails, beet salad, herbal supplements, and extra-virgin olive oil and lemon juice to your menu plan.

THE GALLBLADDER CLEANSE MENU

Breakfast
7:00 a.m. or upon rising: Drink 1 cup hot water with the juice of
¼ lemon and a dash of cayenne pepper
7:10 a.m.: 2 tablespoons extra-virgin olive oil and 1 tablespoon
lemon juice mixed together
7:15 a.m.: Gallbladder Cleanse Cocktail (p. 155)
7:30 a.m.: Choose from the breakfast entrées in Chapter 8 and
include some raw food

Morning program
9:00 a.m.: 1 to 2 teaspoons Beet Salad (p. 147)
9:30 a.m.: 8 ounces of water
10:00 a.m.: Herbal tea with lemon
10:30 a.m.: 8 ounces of water

11:00 a.m.: 1 to 2 teaspoons Beet Salad (p. 147)

11:30 a.m.: 8 ounces of water

Lunch

Noon: Choose from the lunch entrées in Chapter 8 and include some raw food such as a salad or veggie sticks

Afternoon program

1:30 p.m.: 1 to 2 teaspoons Beet Salad (p. 147)

2:00 p.m.: 8 ounces of water

2:30 p.m.: Vegetable juice

3:00 p.m.: 8 ounces of water

3:30 p.m.: 1 to 2 teaspoons Beet Salad (p. 147)

4:00 p.m.: 8 ounces of water

4:30 p.m.: Herbal tea with lemon or fresh vegetable juice

5:00 p.m.: 8 ounces of water

5:30 p.m.: 1 to 2 teaspoons Beet Salad (p. 147)

Dinner

6:00 p.m.: Vegetable juice

Main course salad or dinner entrée of choice; make sure to include some raw food

Supplement: 2 capsules/tablets lipotropic formula

7:15 p.m.: 1 to 2 teaspoons Beet Salad (p. 147)

8:30 p.m.: Chamomile or peppermint herbal tea

Note: *Avoid eating after 7:30 p.m. to give your liver a chance to do its work of cleansing.*

RECIPES FOR GALLBLADDER CLEANSE

Hot Water, Lemon Juice, and Cayenne Pepper

Lemon and cayenne are excellent liver and gallbladder cleansers. Upon rising, squeeze ¼ of a fresh lemon in a cup (8 ounces) of hot water; add a small dash of cayenne pepper and stir.

Extra-Virgin Olive Oil and Lemon Juice

Mix 2 tablespoons extra-virgin olive oil and 1 tablespoon fresh lemon juice in 4 to 6 ounces purified water or juice, which helps to purge the gallbladder gently. Mix vigorously, and drink down quickly. For the gallbladder cleanse, you will be drinking this mixture for seven days.

Gallbladder Cleanse Cocktail

1 handful fresh parsley
4 medium carrots, well scrubbed, end trimmed
2 stalks celery with leaves, ends trimmed
½ lemon, peeled

Bunch up the parsley and push it through the juicer feed tube with the carrots, celery, and lemon. Stir the juice and pour into a glass. Drink as soon as possible to maximize the nutritional value or store in the refrigerator, covered, or take with you in a thermos.

Nutritional analysis: 164 calories (6% from fat) • 1g fat • 6g protein • 39g carbohydrate • >2g dietary fiber • 0mg cholesterol • 205mg sodium

Other Beneficial Fresh Vegetable Juice Combinations

Carrot, beet, and cucumber
Carrot, celery, and endive or kale
Carrot, beet, and coconut milk
Carrot and spinach

If you are sugar sensitive (hypoglycemic or diabetic) and react to carrots or beets, either use smaller amounts than called for or use cucumber and more greens, and flavor with lemon juice or ginger to dilute sugar content. You can also mix in two ounces water.

Lipotropic Formula

Nutritional supplements known as lipotropic formulas containing choline, betaine, and/or methionine and cysteine are designed to promote the flow of fat and bile to and from the liver. They are formulated to improve liver function and enhance detoxification. For the best effect, you will need to get a daily dose of 1,000 mg choline and 1,000 mg of either methionine or cysteine. Take one or two tablets/capsules or more as needed to reach 1,000 mg of choline and methionine or cysteine per day.

THE KIDNEY CLEANSE PROGRAM

When we cleanse the body, it is important to cleanse the kidneys, too. The kidneys are considered a primary organ of elimination. Though they are small, they are so important in our elimination system that we've been given two of them. Under good conditions the kidneys have significant work to do. Most Americans overtax their kidneys by consuming the standard American diet (SAD). When the intestinal tract becomes overwhelmed with toxins and waste, the kidneys are forced to handle the excess. People who are on low-carb diets with a high intake of animal proteins are particularly taxing their kidneys.

During cleansing, the kidneys must process more toxic substances than normal. A number of herbs are helpful in strengthening and toning the kidneys. They facilitate an increase in urine flow, reduce inflammation, and remove uric acid and other crystalline formations. The kidney cleanse program contains a number of natural food and herbal diuretics that not only support the kidneys but also help to rid the body of old stored water, which can facilitate a reduction in facial puffiness and edema. Cucumber, cantaloupe with seeds, asparagus, lemon, kiwifruit, and parsley are all considered natural diuretics.

For seven days, follow the 14-Day Wrinkle Cleanse Diet and include the elements of the kidney cleanse menu plan that includes kidney tonics, cranberry water, and herbal tea.

THE KIDNEY CLEANSE MENU

Breakfast

7:00 a.m. or upon rising: Drink one cup of herbal tea such as agrimony, marshmallow, juniper, or buchu. (These are all diuretic herbs that will help you get rid of excess water and can benefit the urinary tract.)

7:15 a.m.: Fresh juice such as Kidney Tonic (p. 159) or cranberry water

7:30 a.m.: Choose from the breakfast entrées in Chapter 8, and include some raw food

Morning program

9:00 a.m.: 8 ounces cranberry water

10:00 a.m.: Nettle tea with lemon, kidney herbal supplement (see Resources, p. 250), optional

10:30 a.m.: 8 ounces of water

11:00 a.m.: Cranberry water

11:30 a.m.: 8 ounces of water

Lunch

Noon: Choose from the lunch entrées in Chapter 8, and include some raw food such as a salad or veggie sticks

Afternoon program

1:00 p.m.: 8 ounces of water

2:00 p.m.: Cranberry water

Kidney herbal supplement, optional

3:00 p.m.: 8 ounces water or sparkling mineral water with lemon

4:00 p.m.: Cranberry water or nettle tea with lemon

4:30 p.m.: 8 ounces water

5:00 p.m.: Fresh vegetable juice

Dinner

6:00 p.m.: Choose from the dinner entrées in Chapter 8 and include some raw food

8:00 p.m.: Herbal tea with lemon and herbal supplement, optional

Note: *Avoid eating after 7:30 p.m. to give your kidneys a chance to do its work of cleansing.*

RECIPES FOR KIDNEY CLEANSE

Kidney Tonic

1 cucumber (peeled, if not organic)
Handful fresh parsley
1 stalk celery, with leaves, end trimmed
¼ lemon, peeled, or handful of fresh mint
½-inch piece fresh ginger root

Cut the cucumber in half and juice. Bunch up the parsley and juice followed by the celery, lemon or mint, and ginger. (Parsley and celery are kidney tonic juices and natural diuretics.)

Makes 1 serving

Nutritional analysis: 100 calories (10% from fat) • 1g fat • 5g protein • 21g carbohydrate • >2g dietary fiber • 0mg cholesterol • 81mg sodium

Cranberry Water

Cranberry juice is cleansing for the kidneys and good medicine for the urinary tract. I don't recommend the commercially bottled cranberry juices because they contain sweeteners, which are not part of the Wrinkle Cleanse program. You can make your own with pure unsweetened cranberry concentrate (1 to 2 teaspoons, to taste) and water to which you may add a pinch of stevia or a drop or two of Lo Han Guo (see p. 69) or birch sugar (xylitol). Cranberry concentrate can be purchased at health food stores.

Nettle Tea

The herb nettle is used traditionally for kidney cleansing and support and it helps eliminate uric acid. Drink one to two cups of this tea each day; lemon improves the flavor.

THE NEXT STEP

Now that you've completed the cleansing boost programs, you should feel light, clear, and energized. You may be hearing comments about how good you look—like that you're more vibrant, younger looking, and glowing. Some may ask what happened to your wrinkles and lines and ask you if got an eye lift or a face-lift. Now, the key to an effective cleansing program and to maintaining your new you is coming out on the other side with new and improved eating habits and life choices.

By now you've learned the secret to preventing burnout and promoting optimum health. This is the true secret to antiaging. You can return to the cleansing programs whenever you feel sluggish, tired, run down, or notice wrinkles creeping back again. It is advisable to cleanse your body at least once a year; subsequent cleansing programs don't need to be as long as the first one. A couple of weeks in the spring and fall are ideal to prevent premature aging and disease.

The final step, which is Step 4 in the program, follows in Chapter 7. It outlines the nutritional supplements you can use to boost your Wrinkle Cleanse program from start to finish and continue through maintenance. These are the nutrients that can help you maintain your "new you" for life.

Step 4: Vitamins and Minerals That Fight Aging

Step 4, which outlines the vitamins and minerals that fight aging, can be incorporated into all three steps of the Wrinkle Cleanse program. These are the nutrients that we need to protect our body from the damaging effects of oxidative stress (free radical attack), to bind to toxins rendering them harmless, repair damaged collagen, and address numerous other factors that contribute to aging.

Vitamins and minerals are elements that are essential to life. They are known as *micronutrients* because they are needed in relatively small amounts in comparison to the *macronutrients*—carbohydrates, proteins, and fats. Vitamins and minerals act as *coenzymes,* partners with enzymes, which are catalysts or activators in numerous chemical reactions that take place continuously in our body. Some micronutrients—vitamins C and E, selenium, and beta- and alpha-carotene (substances that inhibit the destructive effects of oxidation)—have other functions besides acting as antioxidants and helping form and maintain bones, and some, such as vitamin D, function as hormones.

As we age, we tend to experience more free radical reactions in our body, which accelerate wrinkling and other aspects of aging and precipitate degenerative disease. With each passing year, we have a greater need for antioxidants and other nutrients to help our body neutralize free radicals and other toxic substances, repair damaged tissue, and maintain bodily functions.

It is difficult to get all the nutrients we need just from the food we eat. Our soil is depleted of minerals due to poor farming practices and the use of chemical fertilizers. Fruits and vegetables are often picked too early and don't have a chance to produce the vitamins they would if picked ripe. Seeds are hybridized and weaker than in past generations, which results in plants with fewer nutrients. Add to the mix pesticides, chemical fertilizers, industrial toxins, a stressful lifestyle, limited rest and relaxation, more demands on time and energy, less time to prepare healthful food, consumption of more processed food, and poor dietary choices—and we have a setup for an extraordinary need for supplemental nutrients.

Nutrient supplementation is not optional for most of us—it's imperative. This is why I recommend freshly made vegetable juices and a variety of nutritional supplements as part of the Wrinkle Cleanse.

You should start with a multivitamin and multimineral supplement and then add other supplements as desired. Multivitamins combine a number of nutrients in one capsule or tablet and may supply enough of some vitamins such as A and D and minerals such as chromium and iron to meet your daily needs. Few multivitamin capsules will contain enough vitamin C or B vitamins to meet the needs of a stressful, busy lifestyle. And very few contain nutrients such as alpha lipoic acid or L-carnitine to support your antiaging plan.

If you purchase a high-quality multiformula that provides a wide variety of vitamins and minerals, you can then add other nutrients tailored to your needs and the recommendations for the Wrinkle Cleanse. A "high-quality formula" refers to the material that the nutrients are derived from, that comes from natural sources rather than synthetic. Choose natural sources whenever you can. Look for a good quality supplement at your health food store; you probably won't find quality in a discount store.

Following are the individual nutrients found to be most helpful in preventing or reversing wrinkles and other aspects of aging, along with improving overall health.

ALPHA LIPOIC ACID

Lipoic acid (also known as thioctic acid) is an antioxidant, vitamin-like substance that has similar effects in the body as vitamins C and E. It is a potent free radical scavenger and is effective against both water-soluble and fat-soluble free radicals, making it effective in fighting free radicals in any part of the cell and between cells. It is vital in the production of cellular energy (ATP) and is involved in the conversion of carbohydrates to energy.

Alpha lipoic acid can improve a cell's energy level, or metabolism, which is key to cleansing and antiaging. A higher energy level means cells can remove waste more efficiently and take in nutrients and repair damage more effectively. When a cell's metabolic function is low, it doesn't have the energy to complete these functions, which becomes a telltale sign of aging.

Alpha lipoic acid can also prevent inflammation, which is a major contributor to wrinkles and other signs of aging. It prevents the action of chemicals that damage cells. It can also turn on production of substances that digest damaged collagen, thus reversing wrinkles and scars. Alpha lipoic acid (along with a diet that eliminates sugar) helps prevent sugar from attaching to collagen proteins, which causes sagging and stiff, inflexible skin.

Food sources of alpha lipoic acid are liver and nutritional yeast. The recommended dosage of supplemental alpha lipoic acid is 20 to 50 mg daily.

CAROTENES AND VITAMIN A

Vitamin A is important for the healthy functioning of the immune system and formation of epithelial tissue, which is found throughout the body in the skin, glands, mucous membranes, the lining of hollow organs, and along the respiratory, gastrointestinal, and genito-urinary tracts. Studies indicate that vitamin A promotes cell growth and is essential for healthy skin and eyes. Vitamin A, which is fat soluble, is found only in animal products, and is especially high in fish oils. The best food sources for vitamin A are cod liver oil and fish such as salmon, cod, halibut, whitefish, and swordfish. I recommend that you take a tablespoon of cod liver oil daily (flavored oil is available) and eat fresh wild-caught fish several times a week. I don't recommend you take extra vitamin A supplementation beyond what's in a multivitamin capsule (usually between 2,500 and 5,000 IU) as it is fat soluble and can easily build up in your system, which can result in toxicity if ingested in amounts over 50,000 IU over a period of several years.

Carotenes, such as alpha- and beta-carotene, are converted to vitamin A as needed by the body, and they will not build up in the system. They are found in brightly colored fruits and vegetables such as carrots, collard greens, kale, sweet potatoes, parsley, spinach, Swiss chard, beet greens, chives, butternut squash, watercress, mangos, bell peppers (red is the highest), cantaloupe, endive, apricots, and broccoli. Carotene's most important antiaging functions include:

- Enhancing immune function
- Detoxifying carcinogens
- Scavenging singlet oxygen (free radicals)
- Protecting the skin; acting as natural sun blockers

It is most effective to obtain beta-carotene from your food, which offers its most absorbable form. Get five to nine servings per day of brightly colored, organically grown vegetables and fruit. I suggest that you drink ten to twelve ounces of vegetable juice every day (three-quarters cup juice equals one serving).

(*Note:* Carotenes are very susceptible to oxidative damage; therefore, exposure to air and light can destroy them quickly. It is best to drink carotene-rich juices as quickly as possible or store them in opaque containers, covered, in the refrigerator or a thermos, for not more than twenty-four hours.)

COENZYME Q_{10}

CoQ_{10}, also known as ubiquinone, is an essential part of the mitochondria—the little energy furnaces of our cells. It is involved in the production of ATP, the energy medium of our body processes—and acts as the spark in our body that gets us going. As an antioxidant, CoQ_{10} protects the body against lipid peroxidation. It works with vitamin E to prevent damage to lipid (fat) membranes and plasma lipids. In addition to boosting free radical defense, CoQ_{10} helps fuel production of new collagen, reduce inflammation, and helps improve overall texture and appearance of the skin.

Coenzyme Q_{10} is found in all plant and animal cells. It has been noted that plasma levels of CoQ_{10} are considerably higher (more than double) in vegetarians than in omnivores, indicating that a high intake of plant foods may preserve high CoQ_{10} levels. Recommended dosage of CoQ_{10} is from 100 to 200 mg daily.

ENZYMES AND BETAINE HCL

Digestion of food and assimilation of nutrients are as important as eating high-quality protein, carbohydrates, and fats. Modern methods of food preparation destroy most of our foods' enzymes, requiring the body to provide all the enzymes necessary for digestion. By replacing enzymes lost in cooking through appropriate enzyme supplementation, better digestion can be achieved with minimal stress on the body.

Enzyme supplements should contain protease, amylase, and lipase. Protease is the enzyme that breaks down protein into amino acids. Proper protein digestion is necessary to build and repair tissue and regulate the body's water balance. Amylase breaks down starch and other complex carbohydrates into simple sugars, which is necessary to provide immediate sources of energy and support many other tasks such as normal gallbladder function. Lipase breaks down fats into fatty acids, which is necessary to maintain resilience and lubrication of all cells and tissues and for absorption and transport of essential vitamins. The recommended basic dosage of enzymes is: protease, 20,000 HUT; lipase, 150 LU; amylase, 7,000 DU.

In addition to obtaining plenty of enzymes to aid digestion, we also need adequate gastric acid secretion to break down food in the stomach. Studies indicate that stomach acid secretions decrease with age. Low stomach acidity can cause indigestion. If you have symptoms such as bloating, belching, burning, or gas after a meal or if you have weak, peeling, or cracking fingernails, this may be a sign that you may have low stomach acidity. A test known as the Heidelberg gastric analysis can confirm if this is true (many holistic doctors can perform such a test). An at-home practical test to determine if you may need gastric acid supplementation is by taking hydrochloric acid supplements (betaine HCl) and observing the results such as improvement in digestion and the strength of your nails and hair. Start with one capsule taken in the middle of a meal and work your way up one capsule at a time to three or four with a meal, or until you feel some warmth after you take them. Remember, even the best food is only as good as what we can digest and assimilate. We are not only we eat; we are what we can utilize. The recommended dosage of betaine HCl is 520 mg to start (increase one capsule at a time to three or four with meals, or as directed by your health-care advisor). You may also benefit by adding 20 mg of pepsin.

SILICON

Silicon is the most abundant mineral on earth. It is an essential nutrient that is required for the health and strength of the skin, hair, fingernails, ligaments, tendons, and bones. It also aids the formation of collagen in connective tissues and glucosamine formation. It is necessary for flexible arteries, and plays a major role in preventing cardiovascular disease. Silicon counteracts the effects of aluminum on the body, making it an important mineral in the prevention of Alzheimer's disease. It is also important in preventing osteoporosis in connection with calcium, boron, magnesium, and vitamin K.

A deficiency of silicon can cause dull, brittle, prematurely graying hair, thinning, fragile skin, cracked, brittle nails, and weak bones. In one study, fifty women who showed visible signs of aging in their facial skin, hair, and nails, applied topical silicon (colloidal silicic acid) twice a day and ingested supplemental silicon as colloidal silicic acid (10 ml) daily. Within ninety days, they showed significant signs of improvement in the thickness and strength of their skin, diminished wrinkles, and healthier hair and fingernails. Ultrasound examination showed an increase in the thickness of the dermis (the layer of connective tissue beneath the epidermis—the outermost layer of skin).

Silicon is known as one of nature's great beauty nutrients. Unfortunately, it's content in the aorta, thymus, and skin has been shown to decline with age. Therefore, it is important to include plenty of silicon-rich foods and juices. Though silicon supplementation appears to be safe, the best source is vegetables and fruit. Therefore, I recommend supplementing your diet with fresh vegetable juices and consuming an abundance of silicon-rich foods as much as possible. You could include a small amount of silica or silicic acid supplement to boost your intake. Foods richest in silicon include cucumbers, bell peppers, alfalfa sprouts, beets, brown rice, horsetail grass (an herb), green leafy vegetables, root vegetables (especially parsnips), oatmeal, and whole grains.

The cucumber skin is particularly rich in silicon. The whole cucumber makes a great addition to almost any vegetable juice combination. Unfortunately, most commercially grown cucumbers are sprayed with pesticides and waxed, which is undesirable for our health, and means they need to be peeled. To avoid these chemicals entirely, it is best to purchase organically grown cucumbers. (English cucumbers usually are not waxed.) Drinking the Super Energizer Cocktail (see p. 175) with cucumber in the morning can help your skin become thicker, smoother, younger-looking, and less fragile.

Parsnip juice is also known as a traditional remedy for beautifying the skin, hair, and nails. (See Beautiful Skin Solution for how to combine parsnips with other juices, p. 177.) Adding a cup of nettle tea, which is also rich in silicon and is known to purify the blood and cleanse the kidneys, may also help you look younger. Nettle juice can be used as a hair rinse to help restore color.

Supplemental silicon is available in several different forms: Horsetail (an herb) is rich in silicon. Supplements can be found as silica, sodium metasilicate, and colloidal silicic acid. Typically, dosages range from 5 to 20 mg and should not exceed 50 mg daily.

Keep Your Bones Young

In the end, we may only be as young as our bones. Without strong bones, we will age quickly. Osteoporosis can sneak up on us without symptoms and a fracture could end our life prematurely. Many people are not aware that it takes a lot more than calcium to keep the bones young. Here's the recipe for youthful bones for life.

- Eat plenty of dark leafy greens such as kale, collards, salad greens, parsley, and watercress; they are rich in bone-strengthening nutrients (see p. 168)
- Eat plenty of silicon-rich foods
- Vitamin D: 800 IU per day
- Calcium: 1,000 mg per day for premenopausal women; 1,500 mg for postmenopausal women
- Magnesium: 400 to 800 mg per day
- Vitamin K: 200 to 500 mg per day (if you take Coumadin don't exceed 150 mg)
- Thirty minutes of sunshine per day
- Weight-bearing exercise
- Weight training

SULFUR

A mineral that is part of the chemical structure of methionine, cysteine, taurine (amino acids), and glutathione (an antioxidant), sulfur is found in hemoglobin and all body tissues and is required for the synthesis of collagen and maintaining skin's elastin. Sulfur disinfects the blood, resists bacteria, and protects the protoplasm of cells. It also protects the body against toxins, aids in oxidation reactions, and stimulates bile secretions in the liver. It has the ability to protect the body against the harmful effects of radiation, pollution, and other environmental toxins, making it an important mineral in slowing down the aging process and extending life.

You can get sulfur from a variety of foods and juices. Foods richest in sulfur include onions, eggs, Brussels sprouts, cabbage, garlic, fish, horsetail (herb), kale, turnips, dried beans, and red meat. (I recommend limiting red meat for reasons previously mentioned.)

VITAMIN C

Renowned for its effects on the immune system and for fighting off infection, vitamin C, also known as ascorbic acid, is a premier antiaging nutrient and water-soluble antioxidant. One of its primary functions is to manufacture collagen—the fibrous protein found in skin, bones, cartilage, tendons, and other connective tissue. Since vitamin C plays an important role in structure, it is vital in keeping the skin from sagging. In vitro (test tube), vitamins C and E have been shown to prevent sugar-induced molecular changes in collagen. In animal studies, vitamin C lowered lipid peroxides, free radicals that cause damage to fats (scientifically referred to as oxidation of plasma lipids, which are fats).

Vitamin C has long been studied for its antioxidant action. Ascorbic acid works in water both inside and outside cells and is the first line of defense against free radical attacks. Its key partners are vitamin E and carotenes and the antioxidant enzymes glutathione peroxidase, catalase, and superoxide dismutase. It is also responsible for regenerating oxidized vitamin E, thus restoring its effectiveness in defending the body from free radical attack.

Vitamin C has been shown to reduce inflammation by arresting the production of arachidonic acid—an unsaturated fatty acid that can lead to inflammation and the formation of wrinkles. Taking just 500 mg of vitamin C daily for two months can lower a marker of inflammation known as CRP by 24 percent.

Used topically as freshly activated L-ascorbic acid and ingested via foods and supplements, vitamin C can protect the skin against UV-light exposure. Ascorbyl palmitate seeps into the skin and controls the body's inflammatory response to UV rays, delivering many times more protection from the sun than can be derived from diet alone. UVA and UVB rays cause oxidative damage to collagen, elastin, proteoglycan, cell membranes, and nuclear constituents, and they destroy vitamin C in the skin. When vitamin C levels are low in the skin, the connective tissue breaks down, which contributes to wrinkles, sagging skin, and even skin cancer. But replenishing vitamin C in the skin through supplements and topical treatment that contains L-ascorbic acid (use once or twice a day or according to directions) has significant antiaging and skin cancer preventative action.

During times of stress, whether emotional, physiological (which includes chemical), or psychological, the urinary system excretes vitamin C at a significantly increased rate, increasing the body's need for extra C. Because the human body does not produce vitamin C, as many animals' bodies do, it must be ingested. Supplementation may be the only way to meet our body's needs to prevent infections and other challenges that contribute to inflammation and the aging process.

Foods richest in vitamin C include: bell peppers, kale, parsley, collard greens, broccoli, Brussels sprouts, mustard greens, watercress, cauliflower, persimmons, red cabbage, strawberries, papaya, spinach, oranges, lemons, grapefruit, cabbage, turnips, asparagus, and mangos. Supplemental vitamin C is needed in greater amounts as we age or when we are under stress or ill. As a general guideline, people under age fifty and who are not ill or experiencing a lot of stress can usually benefit from 1,000 to 2,000 mg per day. People age fifty and over or who are experiencing stress or are ill can often benefit from 3,000 to 5,000 mg of vitamin C per day.

Nutrients for Your Skin

The major contributors of skin problems are chronic inflammation, cell damage, and a compromised skin barrier. Chronic inflammation can be caused by everything from UV light to harsh cleaning products, illness, poor dietary choices, chemicals in skin-care products, and toxins. Boosting your skin's permeable barrier is a key step in preventing further damage. You can prevent the microscopic damage that makes your skin age faster by supporting your skin with vitamins such as C and E and other topical nutrients that feed and protect it. (For product recommendations, see Resources, p. 252.)

VITAMIN E

A fat-soluble antioxidant, vitamin E is incorporated into the fatty portion of cell membranes where it protects cells from free radical attacks and damage from heavy metals such as lead and mercury, chemical compounds, and radiation. Vitamin E protects cells from peroxidation of fatty acids, which is the loss of electrons due to free radical attack. Vitamin E is also effective in supporting immune functions and it protects the thymus gland and white blood cells from free radical damage.

One form of vitamin E, the tocotrienols, most effectively repairs skin damage, prevents free radical attacks on cells, and protects the heart. Tocotrienols are found in plants, especially the seeds. Be aware that tocotrienols are very heat sensitive and are easily destroyed by processing and heat. That's why it's important to eat vitamin E-rich foods in their most natural state.

The richest food sources of vitamin E include: sunflower seeds, almonds, wheat germ, peanuts, cold-pressed extra-virgin olive oil, spinach, butter, oatmeal, bran, asparagus, salmon, and brown rice. Recommended supplementation of vitamin E is between 400 to 800 mg daily; the most effective forms include tocotrienols and gamma tocopherols.

ZINC

Important to more than two hundred zinc-dependent enzymes, this nutrient is implicated in more enzymatic reactions than any other mineral. It is incorporated into every cell in the body and is necessary for the healthy function of many hormones. There is a high concentration of zinc in the skin, and it works synergistically with vitamin A and sulfur to maintain healthy hair. It assists enzymes that digest damaged collagen function properly, and it also helps in rebuilding new collagen. And it is vital for healthy immune function. White spots on the fingernails can indicate zinc deficiency.

The richest food sources of zinc include: oysters, ginger root, pecans, split peas, Brazil nuts, egg yolk, whole wheat, rye, oats, peanuts, lima beans, almonds, walnuts, sardines, chicken, clams, tuna, haddock, and shrimp. The recommended dose for zinc supplementation is between 15 and 20 mg daily.

Wrinkle Cleanse Supplement Recommendations

Alpha lipoic acid	20 to 50 mg
Betaine HCl	520 mg (to start) plus 20 mg pepsin
Coenzyme Q_{10}	100 to 200 mg
Enzymes	protease (20,000 HUT), amylase (7,000 DU), lipase (150 LU)
Silicon (silica, silicic acid)	5 to 20 mg; should not exceed 50 mg per day
Vitamin A	2,500 to 5,000 IU
Vitamin C	1,000 to 2,000 mg; over 50, under stress, or ill, 3,000 to 5,000 mg
Vitamin E	400 to 800 mg
Zinc	15 to 20 mg

8

Recipes for Antiaging

The healthy and delicious recipes in this chapter can help you make your 14-Day Wrinkle Cleanse program and the cleansing boost programs a great success. From great-tasting juice recipes to breakfast, lunch, and dinner, you can dine your way to a younger you.

JUICES

Super Energizer Cocktail

This cocktail is a great morning drink—it's very energizing. It's loaded with antioxidants and is an excellent antiwrinkle combination.

1 cucumber (peeled, if not
organic)
1 handful fresh parsley
4 to 5 medium-size carrots,
scrubbed, green tops removed

1 small beet with tops, scrubbed
1-inch piece fresh ginger root,
peeled
1 stalk celery, with leaves
¼ lemon, peeled

Cut the cucumber in half and run it through the juicer. Then bunch up the parsley, place in the juicer's feed tube, and follow with the carrots and beets. Next add the ginger root, celery, and lemon. Serve immediately or chill, covered, until ready to serve.

Makes 1 to 2 servings

Nutritional analysis (per serving): 123 calories (6% from fat) • 1g fat • 5g protein • 28g carbohydrate • 1g dietary fiber • 0mg cholesterol • 122mg sodium

Garden Cocktail

This could also be called the "salsa cocktail" since it has a lot of the vegetables found in salsa. Tomatoes are known to help remove toxins from the body and are beneficial in cleansing the liver.

1 tomato
¼ green bell pepper
1 garlic clove
4 carrots, scrubbed, green tops
removed

2 stalks celery, with leaves
Dash hot sauce

Cut the tomato into chunks that fit your juicer's feed tube and alternate adding green pepper, garlic, carrots, and celery with tomato. Add a dash of hot sauce to the juice and stir well.

Makes 1 serving

Nutritional analysis (per serving): 175 calories (5% from fat) • 1g fat • 5g protein • 41g carbohydrate • 1g dietary fiber • 0mg cholesterol • 183mg sodium

Beautiful Skin Solution

Cucumber and bell pepper are good sources of silicon and parsnip juice is a traditional skin tonic. Drink one cup of this nutritious juice every day to experience the benefits for your skin, hair, and nails.

1 cucumber, peeled if not organic
1 medium parsnip
2 to 3 carrots, scrubbed, tops removed
½ lemon, peeled
¼ green pepper

Cut the cucumber and parsnip lengthwise and feed through the juicer followed by the carrots, lemon, and green pepper, alternating lemon and green pepper with carrots.

Makes 1 to 2 servings

Nutritional analysis (per serving): 143 calories (4% from fat) • 1g fat • 3g protein • 34g carbohydrate • 1g dietary fiber • 0mg cholesterol • 40 mg sodium

The Feel-Good Cocktail

Fennel juice has been used as a traditional tonic to help release endorphins, those "feel-good" peptides, from the brain into the bloodstream. Endorphins help create a mood of euphoria and help dampen anxiety and fear. And there's nothing like a great outlook on life to make us feel younger!

½ Granny Smith or pippin apple
4 medium carrots, scrubbed, tops removed
3 fennel stalks (leaves and flowers are fine to include)
1 stalk celery, with leaves

Juice all ingredients, stir, and serve.
Makes 1 to 2 servings

Nutritional analysis (per serving): 242 calories (4% from fat) • 1g fat • 7g protein • 58g carbohydrate • 1g dietary fiber • 0mg cholesterol • 273mg sodium

Sweet Dreams Nightcap

A deficiency of calcium and magnesium can cause us to wake up in the middle of the night and not be able to drift off to sleep again. Parsley, carrot, and celery are good sources of these minerals. This nightcap also contains some of the B vitamins that help promote restful sleep. Romaine lettuce has been observed to have some sedative effects and celery to have calming effects.

2 romaine lettuce leaves, washed
1 small handful parsley, washed
3 to 4 carrots, scrubbed well, tops removed
3 stalks celery, washed

Bunch up the lettuce and parsley and tuck them into the juicer's feed tube and juice with the carrots and celery. Stir the juice and serve.

Makes 1 to 2 servings

Nutritional analysis (per serving): 178 calories (4% from fat) • 2g fat • 15g protein • 34g carbohydrate • 1g dietary fiber • 0mg cholesterol • 170mg sodium

SMOOTHIES

Very Berry Smoothie

Berries are rich in catechins, phytochemicals that support the immune system and help lower cholesterol. This smoothie is just as delicious if it is made with just one type of berry. If you have only one of the berries on hand, use 1½ cups.

½ cup almond, coconut, or rice milk
½ cup fresh or frozen blueberries
½ cup fresh or frozen blackberries
½ cup fresh or frozen raspberries
½ cup raw cashews
1 scoop protein powder (optional)
6 ice cubes

Place all the ingredients in a blender and process on high speed until smooth. Drink immediately.

Makes 1 serving

Nutritional analysis (per serving): 591 calories (46% from fat) • 32g fat • 13g protein • 72g carbohydrate • 15g dietary fiber • 0mg cholesterol • 25mg sodium

Strawberry-Coconut Smoothie

A quick breakfast when you're on the go, this smoothie is low in carbs and high in nutrition. (Certain brands of coconut milk are lower in carbs than others; a 13.5-ounce can of coconut milk, without all the fillers, should be only 7 grams of carbs.)

10 to 12 ice cubes
1 13.5-ounce can coconut milk
1 cup strawberries
1 scoop protein powder
  (optional)

1 tablespoon flaxseed
1 teaspoon pure vanilla extract
¼ teaspoon almond extract
¼ teaspoon stevia powder (or
  equivalent sweetener)

Place all the ingredients in a blender and process at high speed until well combined. You may add more or less ice, depending on how cold you want your smoothie.

Makes 2 servings

Nutritional analyis (per serving, without protein powder): 372 calories (85.8% from fat) • 32g fat • 4g protein • 8g carbohydrate • 4g dietary fiber • 0mg cholesterol • 27mg sodium

BREAKFAST RECIPES

Green Chili Egg Scramble

This dish is nice served with sliced fresh tomatoes.

1 tablespoon virgin coconut oil
3 tablespoons minced onion
2 tablespoons diced red bell
  pepper
4 eggs

1 tablespoon milk (almond or
  rice milk can be substituted)
1 4-ounce can diced green
  chilies, drained
Salt and pepper to taste

1. Melt the coconut oil in a small skillet over low heat and sauté the onions and red pepper for about 5 minutes, or until onions are translucent and red pepper is tender.
2. While onions are sautéing, whip the eggs with the milk and pour over the onion and red pepper; stir occasionally until mixture is set.
3. Stir in chilies and cook for another minute. Add salt and pepper to taste.

Makes 2 servings

Nutritional analysis (per serving): 160 calories (53% from fat) • 9g fat • 12g protein • 7g carbohydrate • 1g dietary fiber • 374mg cholesterol • 114mg sodium

Fluffy Cheese Omelet

Start with this basic omelet and you can add fillings of your choice such as chopped fresh tomatoes, fresh basil, grilled vegetables, spinach, or artichoke hearts.

4 large eggs
2 tablespoons heavy cream
Freshly ground black pepper
2 tablespoons virgin coconut oil
¼ cup grated or crumbled goat, feta, or cheese of choice

1. In a medium bowl, whisk together eggs, cream, and black pepper. Set aside.
2. In a 10-inch nonstick skillet, melt the coconut oil over medium-high heat. When the oil is hot and bubbly, add the egg mixture, reduce heat to medium and cook, lifting edges to allow uncooked egg to seep underneath.
3. When the bottom layer of egg is cooked but the top is still moist, sprinkle the cheese over one half of omelet and gently fold omelet in half. Cook half a minute longer.
4. Slide the omelet onto a plate and serve immediately.

Makes 2 servings

Nutritional analysis (per serving): 357 calories (81.7% from fat) • 33g fat • 15g protein • 2g carbohydrate • 0g dietary fiber • 409mg cholesterol • 204mg sodium

Mediterranean Frittata

~~~~~~

This frittata will also make a nice dinner entrée served with a salad. The mixture of vegetables offers plenty of carotenes and vitamin C.

1½ tablespoons virgin coconut oil or extra-virgin olive oil

2 small cooked new red potatoes, cubed

2 teaspoons minced fresh thyme or ½ teaspoon dried

1 teaspoon minced fresh rosemary or ¼ teaspoon dried

1 cup water-packed artichoke hearts, quartered

1 small sweet red bell pepper, chopped

Sea salt and freshly ground black pepper, to taste

6 eggs, beaten

¾ cup crumbled feta cheese (dairy or goat)

1. In a large skillet, heat half the oil over low heat. Add the potatoes, thyme, and rosemary and sauté about 10 minutes, or until potatoes become crispy. Add the artichokes, red bell pepper, and salt and pepper to taste. Sauté for 5 minutes, or until vegetables are tender. Remove the vegetables and set aside.

2. In the same skillet, heat the remaining oil, add the eggs and stir slightly, then allow the eggs to set on the bottom, 3 to 4 minutes; the top should still be moist.

3. Spread the vegetable mixture over the top of the eggs and top with the feta cheese. Reduce the heat to low, cover, and cook for about 4 minutes, or until the cheese has melted and the eggs have cooked completely and the bottom of the frittata is golden. (If your skillet is

ovenproof, you could also put it under the broiler for 2 to 3 minutes until the cheese is melted and sizzling.)

Makes 4 servings

Nutritional analysis (per serving): 234 calories (49% from fat) • 13g fat • 15g protein • 15g carbohydrate • 4g dietary fiber • 306mg cholesterol • 440mg sodium

Eggs Benedict Florentine

~~~~~

Serve with Easy Hollandaise Sauce and without the traditional English muffin. You can substitute turkey ham (nitrate-free) or crab cakes for the spinach.

> 2 10-ounce packages frozen chopped spinach
> 1 tablespoon white vinegar
> 8 large eggs
> Easy Hollandaise Sauce (recipe follows)

1. In a medium saucepan, bring water to a boil and cook the spinach until tender. Drain and pat dry with paper towels. Set aside.
2. While the spinach is cooking, in a deep skillet, bring 2 inches of water and the vinegar to a boil over high heat. Reduce heat to a simmer.
3. Crack an egg into a small bowl and tip gently into the simmering water. Repeat with all eggs. Cover the skillet and cook: 3 minutes for soft yolks, 5 minutes for firmer yolks.
4. Using a slotted spoon, remove the eggs from the water and drain thoroughly.

5. Place a heaping serving spoon of spinach for each egg on a plate (2 per plate) and flatten with the spoon; top each spinach mound with a poached egg and Easy Hollandaise Sauce.

Makes 4 servings

Nutritional analysis (per serving): 183 calories (50% from fat) • 10g fat • 16g protein • 27g carbohydrate • 4g dietary fiber • 425mg cholesterol • 231mg sodium

EASY HOLLANDAISE SAUCE

This hollandaise sauce is very easy to make in a blender, and it is so delicious.

3 large egg yolks, whole
2 tablespoons fresh lemon juice
1 dash cayenne pepper
4 ounces (½ cup; 8 tablespoons) unsalted butter, melted and bubbling hot

1. In a blender, combine the egg yolks, lemon juice, and cayenne pepper and blend on high speed for 3 seconds.
2. Remove the lid and, with the motor running, slowly pour hot butter in a steady stream over the eggs. When the butter is all poured in, blend an additional 5 seconds. Taste and adjust seasonings.
3. Serve immediately or keep sauce warm by placing blender in a bowl of warm water.

Makes ¾ cup or 12 tablespoons;
6–12 servings (1 to 2 tablespoons per serving)

Nutritional analysis (per tablespoon serving): 83 calories (94.8% from fat) • 9g fat • 1g protein • trace carbohydrate • trace dietary fiber • 74mg cholesterol • 3mg sodium

SOUPS AND SALADS
(Lunch or Dinner)

French Tomato-Basil Soup

This tomato soup has a very flavorful twist and the added health benefits of parsley and basil. Parsley is one of the most nutritious herbs, rich in vitamin C, chlorophyll, iron, beta-carotene, and bioflavonoids.

1 to 2 tablespoons coconut oil
1 to 2 large onions, finely chopped
1 clove garlic, chopped
4 to 6 vine-ripened tomatoes, chopped
1 tablespoon tomato puree
2 to 3 strips lemon rind, chopped
3 to 4 cups vegetable broth or water
2 tablespoons chopped fresh basil, or 1 teaspoon dried basil
1 teaspoon finely chopped fresh parsley
1 teaspoon chopped fresh thyme or ¼ teaspoon dried thyme
Celtic salt and pepper to taste
Fresh parsley or basil to garnish

1. In a large stockpot or Dutch oven, melt the coconut oil and add the onion and garlic. Cook over low heat for 5 to 6 minutes, until tender and golden brown. Add the remaining ingredients. Bring to a boil, then reduce heat to low and simmer for 20 minutes or until the tomatoes are tender.
2. Let the soup cool, then blend in electric blender or food processor for several minutes. Reheat and serve hot. Garnish with parsley or basil.

Makes 6 to 8 servings

Nutritional analysis (per serving): 83 calories (19% from fat) • 2g fat • 3g protein • 15g carbohydrate • 2g dietary fiber • 1mg cholesterol • 657mg sodium

Mushroom-Barley Soup

~~~~~~

This is a hearty soup loaded with vegetables that makes a great lunch or dinner with a green salad.

4 cups water
¾ cup uncooked medium pearl
  barley
1 tablespoon virgin coconut oil
  or butter
4 medium onions, chopped
2 celery ribs, chopped
1½ pounds sliced fresh
  mushrooms

6 cups low-salt beef broth or
  vegetable broth
2 cups sliced carrots
1 6-ounce can tomato paste
1 teaspoon Celtic salt or sea salt
½ teaspoon freshly ground black
  pepper
½ cup chopped fresh parsley

1. In a large stockpot or Dutch oven, bring the water to a boil and add the barley. Reduce the heat, cover, and simmer for 30 minutes, or until the barley is partially cooked. Do not drain.

2. While the barley is cooking, melt the oil or butter in a Dutch oven and sauté the onions and celery about 5 minutes, or until tender. Add the mushrooms and sauté another 5 minutes, stirring occasionally. Stir in the broth, carrots, tomato paste, and barley with its cooking liquid.

3. Bring to a boil over medium heat, reduce, and cover. Simmer for about 30 minutes, stirring occasionally. Add salt and pepper and adjust seasoning to taste. Garnish with parsley or basil and serve.

Makes 10 servings

Nutritional analysis (per serving): 212 calories (6% from fat) • 2g fat • 16g protein • 40g carbohydrate • 9g dietary fiber • 0mg cholesterol • 628mg sodium

Hearty Split Pea Soup

A thick, nourishing soup, this split pea is loaded with vegetables and herbs. Split peas are good sources of zinc, as are potatoes, carrots, garlic, and thyme.

2 teaspoons virgin coconut oil
1 large yellow onion, chopped
3 large garlic cloves, minced
2 cups dried split peas, washed
  and picked over
2½ quarts water or vegetable
  stock
1 tablespoon vegetable base or
  2 vegetable bouillon cubes
1 medium red potato, diced
1 cup chopped carrots

1 cup chopped celery
1 tablespoon chopped fresh
  basil or 1 teaspoon dried basil
1 tablespoon chopped fresh
  thyme or 1 teaspoon dried
  thyme
1 teaspoon dried marjoram
½ teaspoon dried oregano
½ teaspoon dried tarragon
Sea salt or Celtic salt and freshly
  ground black pepper to taste

1. Heat the oil in a large stockpot or Dutch oven, and sauté the onion and garlic for 5 minutes. Add the split peas and water or vegetable stock and vegetable base or bouillon and bring to a boil. Reduce the heat, cover, and simmer for 1 hour.

2. Add the vegetables and herbs and simmer for another 30 minutes, stirring occasionally. Stir in the salt and pepper as desired.

3. If you like a creamy split pea soup or you want it thicker, you can put all or part of this soup in a blender or food processor and purée. (Puréeing carrot with the other ingredients may produce an undesirable color. If blending, you may want to cook the carrots separately and add them later or omit them.) Serve hot.

Makes 8 servings

Nutritional analysis (per serving): 194 calories (4% from fat) • 1g fat • 13g protein • 35g carbohydrate • 14g dietary fiber • <1mg cholesterol • 49mg sodium

Lima Bean Soup

~~~~~~

This hearty soup, when combined with a savory muffin and garden salad, makes a very satisfying meal. Lima beans were named for the city of the same name in Peru and the beans were discovered in old Peruvian tombs. Dried lima beans have a high protein content and make a good choice for a vegetarian day.

1 cup dried baby lima beans	½ cup chopped green bell pepper
4 cups water or vegetable stock	1 teaspoon fresh basil, or
1 tablespoon virgin coconut oil	½ teaspoon dried basil
1 cup chopped yellow onion	1 28-ounce can stewed tomatoes
1 cup chopped celery	1 teaspoon sea salt or Celtic salt
½ cup chopped carrot	

1. Wash and pick over the beans. Place them in a bowl with enough water to cover them and soak them for 8 hours or overnight.
2. Drain the soaked beans and place them in a large stockpot or Dutch oven with the water or vegetable stock. Cover and bring to a boil. Reduce the heat and simmer until the beans are tender, 1½ to 2 hours.
3. While the beans are cooking, melt the oil in a medium-size skillet and sauté the onion and celery for 5 minutes. Set aside.
4. When the lima beans are tender, add the onion, celery, carrots, bell pepper, basil, and tomatoes. Simmer for about 30 minutes, or until all the vegetables are tender. Add the salt and stir; adjust seasoning to taste and serve.

Makes 4 to 6 servings

Nutritional analysis (per serving): 173 calories (4% from fat) • 1g fat • 9g protein • 35g carbohydrate • 10g dietary fiber • 0mg cholesterol • 421mg sodium

Red Lentil–Spinach Soup

This rosy-colored soup is rich and flavorful. The spinach adds a lot of anti-aging nutrients that include carotenes, vitamin C, iron, and potassium.

1 tablespoon virgin coconut oil
1 cup finely chopped yellow onion
1 cup chopped leeks
3 cloves garlic, minced
1 cup dry red lentils
7 cups water or vegetable broth
1 6-ounce can Italian-style tomato paste

1 vegetable bouillon cube
½ cup tomato juice
1 tablespoon fresh lemon juice
4 cups chopped fresh or frozen spinach, thawed and squeezed in clean tea towel to express excess moisture
Sea salt or Celtic salt and freshly ground pepper to taste

1. Heat the oil in a medium skillet over low heat. Add the onions, leeks, and garlic; sauté until the onions are translucent, about 5 minutes. Set aside.
2. Rinse the lentils in a fine mesh strainer.
3. In a stockpot or Dutch oven, bring the water or vegetable broth to a boil and add the lentils. Skim off any foam that forms on top of lentils. Add the tomato paste, bouillon cube, sautéed onions, leeks, and garlic. Reduce the heat and simmer for 15 minutes.
4. Add the tomato and lemon juice, spinach, and salt and pepper to taste. Simmer for another 15 to 20 minutes, or until lentils are tender.

Makes 6 servings

Nutritional analysis (per serving): 154 calories (5% from fat) • 1g fat • 11g protein • 28g carbohydrate • 12g dietary fiber • 0mg cholesterol • 111mg sodium

Tuscan Sun White Bean Soup

Beans are a good source of fiber, and, like all bean dishes, a good source of protein as well. Add a green salad and you have a complete meal.

1 to 1½ cups dried small white beans, such as navy or great northern
1 tablespoon virgin coconut oil
1 large yellow onion, chopped
4 celery ribs, chopped
4 garlic cloves, minced
6 cups water or vegetable stock
1 tablespoon vegetable base or 2 vegetable bouillon cubes

3 large carrots, chopped
1 cup chopped fresh parsley
2 bay leaves
2 tablespoons chopped fresh oregano or 1½ teaspoons dried oregano
1 teaspoon dried tarragon
Sea salt or Celtic salt and freshly ground black pepper to taste

1. Wash and pick over the beans. Place them in a bowl with enough water to cover and soak them for 8 hours or overnight.
2. Heat the oil in a large stockpot or Dutch oven and sauté the onion, celery, and garlic for about 5 minutes, or until tender. Set aside.
3. Drain the beans and add the water or vegetable stock, the vegetable base or bouillon, and half the carrots, half the parsley, and the bay leaves. Bring to a boil, reduce the heat to medium, cover, and cook 1½ hours or until the beans are tender.
4. When the beans are fully cooked, add the remaining carrots and parsley, the oregano, tarragon, and salt and pepper to taste. Cook for

another 10 to 15 minutes or until the carrots are tender but not mushy. Remove the bay leaves before serving.

Makes 4 to 6 servings

Nutritional analysis (per serving): 218 calories (4% from fat) • 1g fat • 13g protein • 41g carbohydrate • 16g dietary fiber • <1mg cholesterol • 73mg sodium

Gazpacho

3 pounds ripe tomatoes, peeled, seeded, and chopped
½ pound cucumbers, peeled, seeded, and chopped
1 cup chopped celery
½ cup chopped red bell pepper
½ cup chopped red onion
1 teaspoon chopped garlic
1 tablespoon chopped jalapeño pepper

3 tablespoons red wine vinegar
¼ cup extra-virgin olive oil
1½ cups (12 ounces) tomato juice
Salt to taste
Freshly ground black pepper to taste
Dash ground coriander
3 tablespoons chopped cilantro
1 lime, cut into slices

Gazpacho Relish

2 tablespoons small-diced red pepper
2 tablespoons small-diced cucumber
2 tablespoons small-diced red onion
2 tablespoons small-diced red tomatoes

1 teaspoon minced garlic
1 tablespoon lime juice
1 tablespoon extra-virgin olive oil
Celtic salt or sea salt and freshly ground black pepper to taste

1. Combine all the gazpacho ingredients in a blender or food processor, except the lime, and purée until smooth. Transfer to a large bowl and refrigerate for 4 hours.

2. Meanwhile, prepare the Gazpacho Relish by combining all the ingredients.

3. Ladle out chilled soup into pretty bowls, top with a large tablespoon of relish and a slice of lime, and serve.

Makes 8 servings

Nutritional analysis (per serving): 133 calories (55.8% from fat) · 9g fat · 2g protein · 14g carbohydrate · 3g dietary fiber · 0mg cholesterol · 183mg sodium

Basic Garden Salad

There's nothing like a crisp salad with lots of variety—different colors, textures, and flavors. You can start with salad basics such as your favorite greens and add olives, toasted sesame seeds, or goat cheese. You'll need about 6 cups of prepared vegetables and about 6 cups greens to serve four. The vegetables can be either raw or lightly steamed, or you may enjoy a combination of both. Vegetables cook at varying rates; you'll need to steam each type separately or start with the ones requiring longer times and add the others later.

Prepare about 6 cups of torn dark leafy greens. They can be any favorites or a combination of green leaf, romaine, red leaf, butter (bibb), or spring greens (mesclun). Add arugula, watercress, or baby spinach for variety. To this you can add any or all of the following vegetables:

Artichoke hearts (canned or frozen and thawed), rinsed and quartered

Bell peppers (red, green, or yellow), cut into matchsticks 2 to 3 inches long

Carrots, grated or cut into thin matchsticks 2 to 3 inches long

Cherry or grape tomatoes

Corn, fresh or frozen (thawed and drained)

Cucumbers, cut into half moons

Garbanzo beans (chick peas), rinsed and drained

Peas, fresh or frozen (thawed and drained)

Radishes, thinly sliced

Red onion

Scallions

Snow peas, thinly sliced on the diagonal

Sprouts

Summer squash or zucchini, grated or diced into ¼-inch pieces

Lightly steamed (but still crunchy)

Asparagus, cut on the diagonal into 2-inch lengths

Broccoli florets

Cauliflower florets

Green or yellow string beans, snapped into 2-inch lengths

Sugar snap peas

Spicy Chicken Salad

～～～

This main course salad is a delicious way to use leftover chicken. Plan ahead when you make chicken and add some extra to make this salad the next day.

Citrus-Curry Dressing (recipe follows)

2 cups cooked chicken, skin removed, cut into bite-size pieces

3 cups romaine, green leaf, or bibb lettuce, washed, dried, and torn into bite-size pieces

2 cups baby field greens (mesclun)

1 cup chopped cilantro

½ cup chopped red onion

¼ cup chopped green onions

Avocado slices, fresh corn cut from the cob, and toasted sunflower seeds (optional)

1. In a bowl, toss the chicken in half of the Citrus-Curry Dressing to coat. Chill the chicken mixture and remainder of the dressing until ready to use.
2. In a large salad bowl, combine the lettuce and greens, cilantro, and onions. Just before serving, add the chicken and remainder of the dressing and toss.
3. Garnish with sliced avocado, fresh corn cut from the cob, and toasted sunflower seeds, as desired.

Serves 2 as a main course or 4 as a light meal

Nutritional analysis (per serving): 252 calories (42.7% from fat) • 12g fat • 29g protein • 7g carbohydrate • 1g fiber • 69mg cholesterol • 94mg sodium

CITRUS-CURRY DRESSING

3 tablespoons extra-virgin olive oil
3 tablespoons fresh lemon juice
3 tablespoons homemade mayonnaise (p. 196) or commercial*
2 teaspoons healthy low-carb sweetener

1 to 2 teaspoons curry powder
2 tablespoons chopped fresh basil or 1 to 2 teaspoons dried
½ teaspoon sea salt or Celtic salt (optional)

In a small bowl, whisk together all the ingredients.

*If you use commercially made mayonnaise, be aware that many brands use soybean oil or other oils that are not part of this diet.

Homemade Olive Oil Mayonnaise

1 raw free-range egg
1 teaspoon Dijon mustard
1 teaspoon fresh lemon juice
1 cup extra-virgin olive oil (or combination of ½ cup
   olive oil and ½ cup coconut oil)

1. It is extremely important to start with all ingredients at room temperature.
2. In a blender or food processor, combine the lemon juice, mustard, and raw egg.
3. With the motor running, add the oil in a thin, steady stream and process until the mixture is quite thick. The sound in the motor will be an indication of this. If the mixture doesn't thicken, add a bit more oil.

Makes 1 cup (about 16 servings)

Nutritional analysis (per 1 tablespoon serving): 248 calories (79% from fat)
  • 28g fat • 8g protein • trace carbohydrate • trace dietary fiber • 23mg cholesterol
  • 15mg sodium

Spring Greens, Red Onion, and Orange Salad with Curry-Orange Dressing

~~~~~

Fresh orange juice adds flavor and body to the vinaigrette making this a zippy, flavorful salad.

1 cup fresh orange juice
1 small garlic clove, pressed
1 tablespoon apple cider vinegar
1 tablespoon extra-virgin olive oil
1 teaspoon curry powder

¼ teaspoon sea salt or Celtic salt
2 navel oranges
4 cups spring greens (mesclun)
½ red onion, thinly sliced
½ cup toasted slivered almonds

1. In a small saucepan, bring the orange juice to a boil and reduce it to ⅓ cup, about 10 minutes.
2. Transfer the orange juice to a small bowl and whisk in the garlic, vinegar, oil, curry powder, and salt. Set aside.
3. Using a serrated knife, cut the peel from the top and bottom of the oranges. Set on end and remove the outer skin and pith. Cut crosswise into ¼-inch-thick rings. Cut rings in half, and then crosswise in half again.
4. Place the greens, onion, and orange slices in a medium salad bowl and toss with the dressing. Sprinkle slivered almonds on top and serve.

Makes 4 servings

Nutritional analysis (per serving): 220 calories (49% from fat) • 13g fat • 7g protein • 23g carbohydrate • 6g dietary fiber • 0mg cholesterol • 151mg sodium

Caesar Salad

~~~~~

Romaine lettuce is one of the most nutritious of the salad greens, with far more carotenes than its paler cousins, iceberg and Boston.

½ cup extra-virgin olive oil
2 large garlic cloves, crushed or pressed
⅓ cup fresh lemon juice
1 tablespoon red or white wine vinegar
½ teaspoon Dijon mustard
½ teaspoon Worcestershire sauce

¼ teaspoon freshly ground black pepper
¼ teaspoon sea salt or Celtic salt
1 large head romaine lettuce, torn in bite-size pieces
⅓ cup grated Parmesan cheese
¼ cup toasted sunflower seeds

1. To begin preparing the dressing, pour the oil into a small jar, add the garlic, cover, and let stand from 1 to 24 hours. (The longer the garlic soaks, the more garlic flavor the oil will have.)

2. Pour the lemon juice, vinegar, mustard, Worcestershire sauce, salt, and pepper in a blender or food processor. Discard the garlic, and with the blender or food processor running, drizzle in the garlic-flavored olive oil. (This makes about 1½ cups dressing; you may have some left over for another salad. It should last a couple of weeks in a covered container in the refrigerator.)

3. In a large salad bowl, lightly toss the lettuce with a portion of the dressing to coat. Sprinkle the Parmesan cheese and sunflower seeds over top and serve.

Makes 4 servings greens / 1½ cups dressing; 8 servings dressing (1 tablespoon)

Nutritional analysis (per serving): 230 calories (76% from fat) • 21g fat • 7g protein • 6g carbohydrate • 3g dietary fiber • 6.5g cholesterol • 245mg sodium

Lemon-Artichoke Salad

~~~

Artichoke hearts and leaves have a high alkaline content, which is good to balance our highly acidic Western diet. They are also high in fiber and are one of the "liver friendly" foods. Include them also for their carotenes, vitamin C, calcium, and iron.

5 cups romaine lettuce, torn in bite-size pieces
4 Roma or plum tomatoes, quartered
½ 14-ounce can water-packed or frozen, thawed artichoke hearts, quartered
1 2¼-ounce can sliced ripe black olives, drained

3 tablespoons water
3 tablespoons fresh lemon juice
2 garlic cloves, minced or pressed
1 teaspoon sea salt or Celtic salt
1 teaspoon freshly ground black pepper
3 tablespoons extra-virgin olive oil
¼ cup grated Parmesan cheese

1. In a large salad bowl, toss the romaine, tomatoes, artichoke hearts, and olives.
2. In a small bowl, whisk together the water, lemon juice, garlic, salt, and pepper. Slowly drizzle in the olive oil, whisking vigorously to emulsify.
3. Drizzle the dressing over the salad and toss to coat. Sprinkle the Parmesan on top and serve.

Makes 4 servings

Nutritional analysis (per serving): 198 calories (59% from fat) • 14g fat • 6g protein • 16g carbohydrate • 6g dietary fiber • 4mg cholesterol • 830mg sodium

Multigrain Florentine Salad

This salad is a huge hit, whether for family and friends or potluck dinners. But don't just choose it for its great taste. Spinach is a rich source of chlorophyll, a phytochemical that gives plants their green color. Chlorophyll is known to help improve skin texture, purify the blood, and detoxify the body.

1 cup cooked quinoa (see p. 230 for cooking instructions)
1 cup cooked spelt berries (optional)
½ cup cooked brown rice
¾ cup grated carrot
Juice of 1 lemon
1 teaspoon finely chopped lemon peel
3 tablespoons extra-virgin olive oil
2 tablespoons finely chopped fresh basil or 2 teaspoons dried basil
1 large garlic clove, pressed
1 teaspoon honey
Pinch of cayenne pepper
Pinch of sea salt or Celtic salt
1 bunch of fresh spinach, stems removed and torn into bite-size pieces
½ cup chopped pecans, toasted

1. In a large salad bowl, combine the quinoa, spelt, if using, brown rice, and carrot.
2. In a small bowl, whisk together the lemon juice, lemon peel, olive oil, basil, garlic, honey, cayenne, and salt. Pour the dressing over the grain mixture and combine well. Refrigerate until ready to serve. (If the mixture has a chance to marinate for a couple of hours, it will be more flavorful.)
3. Just before serving, gently toss in the spinach. Sprinkle the pecans over top.

Makes 4 servings

Nutritional analysis (per serving): 262 calories (43% from fat) • 13g fat • 7g protein • 32g carbohydrate • 7g dietary fiber • 0mg cholesterol • 64mg sodium

ADDITIONAL SALAD DRESSINGS AND VEGGIE DIPS

Lemon–Olive Oil Dressing

To make this dressing, follow the instructions for the Caesar Salad dressing (p. 198), omitting the Parmesan cheese.

Nutritional analysis (per 2 tablespoon serving): 123.5 calories (96% from fat) • 13.5g fat • trace protein • 1.5g carbohydrate • trace dietary fiber • 0mg cholesterol • 71mg sodium

Lemon-Tarragon Dressing

You can make your own tarragon vinegar for this dressing in just minutes by adding fresh tarragon to white wine vinegar, rice vinegar, or distilled white vinegar. Place about 1 cup of rinsed and dried fresh tarragon in a dry, heatproof jar. Heat two cups of vinegar and pour over herbs, completely covering them. Cap the jar and let the herbs steep for at least 10 days, shaking the jar occasionally. Decant the vinegar, filter or strain it if desired, and store it in a sterilized bottle.

2 tablespoons tarragon vinegar
2 tablespoons extra-virgin
  olive oil
2 teaspoons honey, or low-carb
  healthy sweetener
1 garlic clove, minced

½ teaspoon Celtic salt or sea salt
¼ teaspoon ground mustard
¼ teaspoon freshly ground black
  pepper
¼ teaspoon Worcestershire
  sauce

In a small bowl, whisk together all ingredients. Store leftovers in a capped jar or container in the refrigerator for up to 3 weeks.

Makes about ½ cup

Nutritional analysis (per 2 tablespoon serving): 98 calories (80% from fat) • 9g fat • trace protein • 5g carbohydrate • trace dietary fiber • 0mg cholesterol • 360 mg sodium

Basil-Parmesan Vinaigrette

½ to ¾ cup chopped fresh basil
1 cup extra-virgin olive oil
2 cloves garlic, chopped
1 tablespoon grated Parmesan
  cheese

¼ cup balsamic vinegar
Celtic sea salt and freshly
  ground pepper to taste

Add all ingredients to food processor or blender and process until well combined. Season to taste.

Makes about 1½ cups

Nutritional analysis (per 2 tablespoon serving): 48 calories (80% from fat) • 4.5g fat • trace protein • 2.5g carbohydrate • trace dietary fiber • 0mg cholesterol • 180mg sodium

Asian Dressing

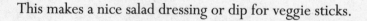

3 tablespoons extra-virgin
olive oil
2 tablespoons tamari or light
soy sauce
2 tablespoons orange juice
2 tablespoons apple cider vinegar

1 tablespoon orange zest
4 large garlic cloves, pressed or
minced
2 teaspoons finely minced fresh
ginger root

Combine all ingredients in a small bowl and whisk until well combined.

Makes about ⅔ cup

Nutritional analysis (per 2 tablespoon serving): 82 calories (86% from fat) • 8g fat •
1g protein • 2g carbohydrate • trace dietary fiber • 0mg cholesterol • 403mg sodium

Salsa

This makes a nice salad dressing or dip for veggie sticks.

1 pound tomatoes, diced
1 medium yellow onion, diced
6 tablespoons chopped fresh
cilantro
2 tablespoons fresh lime juice

1 teaspoon fresh lime zest
2 large garlic cloves, minced
1 large jalapeño, seeded and
minced

Toss all ingredients in a medium bowl until well blended. Refrigerate
until ready for use.

Makes 2 cups; 4½ cup servings

204 • The Wrinkle Cleanse

Nutritional analysis (per serving): 41 calories (3% from fat) • 1g fat • 1.5g protein • 8g carbohydrate • 2g dietary fiber • 0mg cholesterol • 1mg sodium

Hummus

~~~~~~

Hummus makes a very nutritious dip for veggies. And although you can buy commercially made hummus, there's nothing quite like homemade.

1 16-ounce can garbanzo beans (chick peas)
3 tablespoons fresh lemon juice
2 tablespoons extra-virgin olive oil, plus additional for drizzling
½ cup tahini (sesame paste)
¼ cup chopped yellow onion

2 to 3 cloves garlic, pressed
1 teaspoon ground cumin
Dash cayenne pepper
½ teaspoon Celtic salt or sea salt
Chopped fresh parsley and paprika (optional)

1. Drain the garbanzo beans, reserving ¼ cup of the liquid.
2. In a blender or food processor, combine the garbanzo beans, lemon juice, olive oil, tahini, onion, garlic, cumin, cayenne, and salt. Purée until smooth, adding garbanzo bean liquid as needed to thin the mixture.
3. Refrigerate for 3 to 4 hours before serving, to blend flavors. Drizzle a bit of olive oil over top and sprinkle with parsley and paprika, if using.

Makes 5 servings

Nutritional analysis (per 2 tablespoon serving): 529 calories (39% from fat) • 24g fat • 22g protein • 62g carbohydrate • 18g dietary fiber • 0mg cholesterol • 264mg sodium

MAIN COURSES
(Lunch or Dinner Recipes)

Spicy Turkey Tostadas

These tostadas are easy to make and a nutritious version of a fast food dish. On a busy night, this is a quick and delicious meal.

1 tablespoon coconut oil	1 teaspoon chili powder
½ to ¾ pound ground lean turkey	½ teaspoon ground cumin
½ cup chopped onion	½ teaspoon sea salt or Celtic salt
½ cup chopped green bell pepper	½ cup fresh or frozen corn, thawed
2 garlic cloves, minced	8 5-inch corn tortillas
1 16-ounce can refried beans	2 cups torn lettuce pieces
1 16-ounce can black beans, rinsed and drained	½ cup Mexican shredded cheese blend
1 cup Salsa plus extra for dressing, as desired, commercial or homemade (p. 203)	½ cup chopped tomatoes
	½ cup chopped fresh cilantro

1. Heat 1 teaspoon of the oil in a large skillet and cook the turkey over medium heat until there is no pink remaining; drain and set aside.
2. Add the remaining oil and sauté the onion, green pepper, and garlic for 3 to 5 minutes, or until tender.
3. While the onion mixture is cooking, heat the refried beans on low; cover to keep warm.
4. When onion mixture is tender, stir in the black beans, salsa, chili powder, cumin, and salt. Cook for 1 minute and add the cooked turkey and the corn. Cook for 3 minutes.

5. While the onion-turkey mixture is cooking, heat the corn tortillas in the oven or on the stove in a pan brushed with oil.

6. Spread about ¼ cup refried beans on each tortilla and top with about ⅛ of the turkey mixture. Sprinkle a little cheese over the turkey mixture and top with lettuce, tomatoes, and cilantro. You may wish to add extra salsa over top of the greens, as desired.

Makes 4 servings

Nutritional analysis: 526 calories (22% from fat) • 13g fat • 33g protein • 72g carbohydrate • 18g dietary fiber • 51mg cholesterol • 1,600mg sodium

Baked Tilapia with Tarragon-Quinoa Stuffing

Quinoa is a tiny grain with a light airy texture and a slight nutty flavor. It's delicious in stuffing or served as a side dish. For stuffing, it can replace bread crumbs and can be combined with wild rice, brown rice, millet, spelt, or buckwheat. It is one of the best sources of vegetable protein and offers more iron, calcium, and phosphorus than most other grains.

3 tablespoons virgin coconut oil or unsalted butter, plus 1 tablespoon cold unsalted butter

¼ cup thinly sliced scallions (use white and tender light green parts from about 4 scallions)

1 cup cooked quinoa (see p. 230 for cooking instructions)

2 teaspoons chopped fresh tarragon or 1 teaspoon crumbled dried tarragon

1 large egg, beaten

Celtic salt or sea salt and freshly ground black pepper

4 tilapia fillets (or any white fish), rinsed and patted dry, about 6 ounces each
⅓ cup vermouth or white wine

⅓ cup low-salt chicken broth, homemade or commercial
2 teaspoons Dijon mustard

1. Place a rack in the upper third of the oven and preheat to 400°F.
2. Melt 4 tablespoons of coconut oil or butter in a medium saucepan or skillet on medium-low heat. Transfer 1 tablespoon to a small dish and keep warm and lightly brush the inside of a 9 x 13-inch baking dish with some of the melted oil or butter.
3. Add the scallions to the remaining oil or butter in the saucepan and cook, stirring, until softened, for 2 to 3 minutes.
4. In a medium bowl, mix the scallion butter with the quinoa, tarragon, beaten egg, and salt and pepper to taste.
5. Lightly season the fish fillets on both sides with salt and pepper. Lay a fillet on a working surface with the pointed end closest to you. Mound ¼ to ½ cup of the stuffing on the pointed half of the fillet. Fold the wide end of the fillet over and press firmly (don't squish) to cover the stuffing. (A bit of the stuffing will remain exposed.) Put the stuffed fillet in the baking dish. Repeat the procedure with the remaining fillets. Brush the tops of the fillets with the reserved tablespoon of melted oil or butter.
6. Pour the vermouth or white wine and chicken broth into the baking dish, not over the fillets. Bake until the fish feels firm to touch but flaky and the insides of the fillets look opaque when pierced with the tip of a sharp knife, 20 to 25 minutes.
7. Using a thin, flexible slotted metal spatula, transfer the fillets to 4 dinner plates.
8. Add the 1 tablespoon of butter to the hot baking dish and whisk until the butter melts. Add the mustard and whisk until well com-

bined, and season with salt and pepper to taste. Spoon the sauce over the fillets and serve immediately.

Makes 4 servings

Nutritional analysis (per serving): 378 calories (42% from fat) • 17g fat • 36g protein • 13g carbohydrate • 1g dietary fiber • 140mg cholesterol • 520mg sodium

Grilled Mustard-Rosemary Chicken

This chicken is great leftover for Spicy Chicken Salad (p. 194) or sliced and served over a bed of greens or Caesar Salad the next day. You can scale this recipe up or down as needed.

> 3½ to 4 pounds skinless, boneless chicken breasts, rinsed and patted dry
> 1½ teaspoons Celtic salt or sea salt and freshly ground black pepper
> ⅓ cup Dijon mustard
> ⅓ cup mayonnaise, homemade (p. 196) or commercial
> 1 teaspoon chopped fresh rosemary or ½ teaspoon dried rosemary

1. Prepare your grill. If using a gas grill, heat to medium high.
2. Put the chicken in a large bowl and season with salt and ample ground pepper.
3. In a small bowl, combine the mustard, mayonnaise, and rosemary.
4. Spoon the mustard mixture over the chicken and toss to coat all the chicken breasts well. Marinate for 30 minutes.
5. Spread the chicken out on the grill and watch the heat carefully.
6. Cover the grill and cook the chicken on one side for 2 to 3 minutes, or until golden brown and grill marks form. Rotate the chicken 90

degrees and grill another 2 to 3 minutes, which should give you a nice crosshatch of grill marks.

7. Flip the chicken over and repeat until chicken is cooked through with no pink in the center. Total cooking time should be 8 to 12 minutes.
   Makes 8 servings

Nutritional analysis (per serving): 321 calories (39% from fat) • 13g fat • 47g protein • 1.5g carbohydrate • 1g dietary fiber • 130mg cholesterol • 480mg sodium

Red Lentil–Rice Patties with Coconut-Cilantro Sauce

You can make the red lentils and rice ahead of time and store in the refrigerator. The Coconut-Cilantro Sauce is delicious on vegetables as well as the patties. You might want to make extra for the next day.

Cilantro Sauce

- 1 cup cilantro, chopped
- ¼ cup coconut milk
- 2 tablespoons fresh lemon juice
- 1 jalapeño pepper, stemmed and seeded
- 1 small garlic clove
- 1 1-inch piece fresh ginger root
- ½ teaspoon sea salt or Celtic salt

Patties

- 1 cup brown rice
- ½ cup red lentils
- 4 cups water
- ½ teaspoon turmeric
- 1 teaspoon sea salt or Celtic salt
- 2 tablespoons plus 4 teaspoons virgin coconut oil
- 1 teaspoon cumin seeds
- 2 cups finely chopped yellow onions
- ¼ teaspoon red pepper flakes
- ¼ cup arrowroot powder

To make the sauce:

1. Put all the ingredients in a blender or food processor. Purée until smooth and set aside.

To make the patties:

2. Place the rice and lentils in a medium saucepan with water, turmeric, and salt. Cover, bring to a boil, reduce the heat, and simmer for 10 minutes. Remove the cover and simmer, without stirring, for another 20 to 25 minutes, or until the water is absorbed.

3. While the rice and lentils are cooking, heat the 2 tablespoons of oil in a medium skillet over medium-high heat. Add the cumin seeds and cook for 1 minute, stirring frequently. Add the onions and lower heat to medium; cook for about 10 minutes, or until onions are golden. Add the red pepper flakes, stir, and set aside.

4. When rice and lentils are done, place them in a medium bowl and add the onion mixture. Combine well and let stand until cool, about 20 minutes.

5. When the mixture has cooled, spread the arrowroot on a large plate. Form the lentil-rice mixture into 8 patties. Evenly coat each patty on both sides with the arrowroot and set aside until ready to cook.

6. Heat 2 teaspoons of oil in a large skillet over medium-high heat. Cook 4 patties, until golden, about 2 minutes. Then turn and cook the other side 2 minutes or until golden. Remove to a plate and keep warm. Heat the remaining 2 teaspoons of oil and cook the remaining 4 patties. Spoon the Coconut-Cilantro Sauce over the patties and serve warm.

Makes 4 servings

Nutritional analysis for 2 lentil patties (per serving): 317 calories (6% from fat) • 2g fat • 11g protein • 64g carbohydrate • 10g dietary fiber • 0mg cholesterol • 548mg sodium

Nutritional analysis for cilantro sauce (per ¼ cup serving): 50 calories (44% from fat) • 3g fat • 2g protein • 6g carbohydrate • 1g dietary fiber • 0mg cholesterol • 192mg sodium

Baked Flounder

~~~~~~

This is a quick, easy meal when you don't have a lot of time for preparation. Flounder is delicious with this coating, but any white fish can be used.

½ cup cornmeal
1 teaspoon sea salt or Celtic salt
½ teaspoon dried parsley
½ teaspoon paprika
½ teaspoon freshly ground black pepper
1 egg

¼ cup dairy, almond, or rice milk
4 flounder fillets, or any white fish (6 ounces each)
2 teaspoons virgin coconut oil
2 tablespoons grated Parmesan cheese

1. Preheat the oven to 425°F.
2. In a shallow, oblong pan or bowl, combine the cornmeal, salt, parsley, paprika, and pepper. In a shallow bowl, beat egg and milk until well combined.
3. Coat each fillet with the cornmeal mixture, then dip in the egg mixture, and then in the cornmeal mixture again.
4. Melt the oil in a baking pan large enough to accommodate the fillets and arrange the fillets in a single layer. Sprinkle with Parmesan cheese on top and bake for 8 to 10 minutes, or until the fish flakes easily with a fork and is opaque in the center.

Makes 4 servings

Nutritional analysis (per serving): 252 calories (18% from fat) • 5g fat • 35g protein • 15g carbohydrate • 1g dietary fiber • 129mg cholesterol • 734mg sodium

Millet-Walnut Stuffed Peppers

~~~~~

Millet is an ancient grain that makes a great base for stuffing. It was one of the first grains used for food in China, Egypt, India, and Africa. It is still used in Asia and Africa as a staple. Because it is gluten free, it is ideal for those who are sensitive to gluten. It has a chewy texture and a slightly nutty taste. It combines well with vegetables and beans and can be used as a cereal.

½ cup millet, rinsed and drained
1½ cups vegetable broth
4 medium red bell peppers
1 cup fresh or frozen corn, thawed
1 medium yellow onion, finely chopped
½ cup chopped walnuts
2 green onions, finely chopped
1 tablespoon chopped fresh mint or 1 teaspoon dried mint
2 teaspoons finely minced fresh lemon peel or ½ teaspoon dried lemon zest

2 teaspoons fresh chopped oregano or ½ teaspoon dried oregano
1 garlic clove, minced
1 teaspoon sea salt or Celtic salt
½ teaspoon freshly ground black pepper
2 tablespoons virgin coconut oil (melted if solid) or extra-virgin olive oil

1. Preheat the oven to 350°F.
2. Simmer the millet and broth in a medium saucepan until tender and broth is absorbed, 30 to 35 minutes. Transfer the millet to a large bowl and set aside.
3. Cut the tops off the red peppers and remove the seeds and ribs. Parboil in a large saucepan for 3 to 5 minutes. Drain and rinse in cold water; set aside.

4. Fluff the cooked millet with a fork and add the corn, onion, walnuts, green onions, mint, lemon peel, oregano, garlic, salt, and pepper.
5. Spoon ¼ of the millet stuffing into each pepper and drizzle a bit of oil over each pepper. Place in a baking dish brushed with oil and bake for 1 hour, or until tender.

Makes 4 servings

Nutritional analysis (per serving): 275 calories (34% from fat) • 11g fat • 10g protein • 39g carbohydrate • 8g dietary fiber • 0mg cholesterol • 545mg sodium

Grilled Salmon

The marinade with an Asian flair makes this salmon extra special. Wild-caught salmon is a fish to include often in your antiaging diet because it is an excellent source of omega-3 fatty acids.

4 salmon steaks, about 6 ounces each	2 to 3 tablespoons honey or pure maple syrup
¼ cup soy sauce	4 scallions, chopped
¼ cup extra-virgin olive oil	2-inch piece of fresh ginger root, grated

1. Rinse the salmon and pat dry with paper towels. Set aside.
2. In a shallow oblong dish, combine the soy sauce, oil, honey or maple syrup, scallions, and ginger root. Add the salmon and marinate at cool room temperature for 30 to 60 minutes, turning once to marinate on both sides.

3. While the salmon is marinating, prepare the grill. Grill the salmon over medium heat, covered. Grill about 5 to 6 minutes on one side and then turn and repeat until salmon flakes easily when tested with a fork, about another 5 minutes.

   Makes 4 servings

Nutritional analysis (per serving): 367 calories (48% from fat) • 19g fat • 35g protein • 12g carbohydrate • 1g dietary fiber • 88mg cholesterol • 1,146mg sodium

Fish Tacos

If you'd like to try tacos that are healthier and part of the antiwrinkle program, I think you'll enjoy this flavorful version.

1 packet taco seasoning	1½ pounds halibut or cod, cut
3 tablespoons fresh orange juice	into ¾-inch cubes
3 tablespoons fresh lime juice	8 corn tortillas, warmed
1 jalapeño pepper, seeded and	1 papaya, peeled and seeded,
finely chopped	coarsely chopped
¼ cup chopped cilantro	3 cups shredded lettuce

1. Preheat oven to 375°F.
2. In a small bowl, combine 1 tablespoon of the taco seasoning, 1 tablespoon orange juice, 1 tablespoon lime juice, the jalapeño pepper, and cilantro. Cover and refrigerate.
3. In a shallow 2-quart baking dish, combine the remaining orange juice, lime juice, and taco seasoning. Place the fish in the baking dish, cover, and bake for about 15 minutes or until fish flakes easily with a fork.

4. Heat tortillas in oven or skillet brushed with oil. Lay a tortilla on a working surface and place a spoonful of fish in the center. Top with the papaya and shredded lettuce and fold in half. Repeat with remaining tortillas.

Makes 4 servings

Nutritional analysis (per taco): 173 calories (14% from fat) • 3g fat • 20g protein • 17g carbohydrate • 2g dietary fiber • 27mg cholesterol • 381mg sodium

Spicy and Crispy Broiled Halibut

This is a flavorful entrée you can make in less than 30 minutes so it's great for a busy night. Halibut is very rich in iodine and iodine deficiency is related to a sluggish thyroid, which can contribute to weight gain. To maintain a healthy thyroid it's beneficial to eat more fish, seafood, and sea vegetables.

4 halibut steaks, 6 ounces each, or 1½ pounds halibut, cut into 4 pieces, rinsed and patted dry (any white fish can be substituted)
2 tablespoons fresh lemon juice
1 cup mayonnaise, homemade (p. 196) or commercial
⅓ cup finely chopped yellow onion
1 tablespoon Dijon mustard
2 teaspoons Italian herb seasoning
4 dashes Tabasco sauce
Sea salt or Celtic salt and freshly ground black pepper to taste

1. On each side of the fish steak, make 3 diagonal cuts 2 inches long and ½-inch deep. Place the fish in a shallow bowl and pour the lemon juice over the fish, making sure it seeps into the cuts. Let the fish stand in the lemon juice, uncovered, at cool room temperature for

30 minutes. (If you're in a hurry, you don't have to marinate the fish, but it does add flavor.)

2. In a shallow bowl, stir together the mayonnaise, onion, mustard, Italian herb seasoning, and Tabasco sauce. Salt and pepper the fish. Coat both sides of each fish steak with the mayonnaise mixture.

3. Arrange the fish steaks on a broiler pan and spread any remaining mayonnaise mixture over top of fish steaks. Broil for about 5 minutes on each side, or until center is opaque.

Makes 4 servings

Nutritional analysis (per serving): 459 calories (12% from fat) • 5.7g fat • 38g protein • 60g carbohydrate • 1g dietary fiber • 40mg cholesterol • 219mg sodium

Grilled Pepper-Crusted Chicken

Tarragon is an herb that goes well with chicken and adds distinctive flavor to the marinade.

1 3- to 4-pound frying chicken, cut into serving pieces
3 tablespoons extra-virgin olive oil
4 tablespoons fresh lemon juice
2 large garlic cloves, crushed
1 tablespoon cracked black peppercorns
1 tablespoon red pepper flakes
1 tablespoon chopped fresh tarragon or 1 teaspoon dried tarragon
Sea salt or Celtic salt to taste

1. Rinse the chicken and pat dry; set aside.
2. In a large shallow bowl, mix together the remaining ingredients. Add the chicken pieces, tossing to coat thoroughly. Cover and marinate in the refrigerator for 4 hours, turning occasionally.
3. Prepare the grill. When ready, spread the chicken on the grill. Reserve the marinade. Grill the chicken for about 20 to 25 minutes, turning occasionally, and brushing frequently with the marinade until all pieces are crispy brown and cooked thoroughly (no pink in the center and the juices are clear).

Note: Do not brush the chicken with the marinade after you have finished grilling, since raw chicken was previously in the marinade.

Makes 4 servings

Nutritional analysis (per serving): 307 calories (48% from fat) • 16g fat • 36g protein • 3.5g carbohydrate • 1g dietary fiber • 115mg cholesterol • 416mg sodium

Creamed Turkey with Mushrooms

This dish is a special treat and the sauce goes nicely over wild and brown rice. If you have leftover corn bread, this entrée also tastes great spooned over a piece of warmed corn bread.

1½ pounds turkey cutlet, cut into 1-inch pieces (chicken can be substituted)

Sea salt and freshly ground black pepper to taste

2 teaspoons chopped fresh thyme or ½ teaspoon dried thyme

3 tablespoons unsalted butter or virgin coconut oil

2 cups sliced mushrooms
¼ cup minced shallots
⅔ cup dry white wine
⅔ cup chicken broth

⅔ cup heavy cream (coconut milk can be substituted)
Dash nutmeg
¼ cup chopped fresh parsley

1. Season the turkey with salt, pepper, and thyme. Heat 2 tablespoons of butter or oil over medium-high heat in a large skillet. Add the turkey and cook for 3 to 4 minutes, or until golden.
2. Add the mushrooms and cook for 2 to 3 minutes, stirring occasionally. Transfer the turkey mixture to a plate or bowl and keep warm.
3. In the same skillet, melt the remaining butter or oil over medium heat and add the shallots; cook for 2 minutes. Stir in the wine and broth, scraping browned pieces from the bottom of the pan, and bring to a boil. Reduce the heat and simmer for 5 minutes. Add the cream and the nutmeg and simmer for 5 minutes.
4. Return the turkey mixture to the skillet, stir in the parsley, and heat through.

Makes 6 servings

Nutritional analysis (per serving): 266 calories (41% from fat) • 12g fat • 31g protein • 3.5g carbohydrate • 0.7g dietary fiber • 8mg cholesterol • 168mg sodium

SIDE DISHES
(Lunch or Dinner Recipes)

Dressed-up Broccoli

Broccoli is a member of the cruciferous vegetable family, known for their cancer-fighting properties. By itself, broccoli isn't too appealing to many people, but dressed with this vinaigrette it's packed with flavor as well as nutrition.

1 pound broccoli florets
1 teaspoon paprika
1 tablespoon prepared mustard
½ teaspoon sea salt or Celtic salt
Dash of freshly ground black pepper
1 tablespoon pure maple syrup (or equivalent healthy low-carb sweetener)

¼ cup red wine or apple cider vinegar
3 tablespoons extra-virgin olive oil
1 tablespoon chopped olives
1 tablespoon chopped yellow onion

1. Steam the broccoli until tender and bright green; do not overcook.
2. While the broccoli is steaming, mix the remaining ingredients in a small saucepan and heat until warm, stirring frequently.
3. Toss the broccoli and the dressing in a serving bowl and serve hot.
   Makes 6 servings

Nutritional analysis (per serving): 98 calories (65% from fat) • 7.5g fat • 2.5g protein • 7g carbohydrate • 2.5g dietary fiber • 0mg cholesterol • 250mg sodium

Kale with Garlic and Red Pepper

This hearty kale dish is prepared in a simple Italian style and is considered a heart-healthy dish in the Mediterranean diet. Kale is an excellent source of calcium, offering about 250 milligrams of this important mineral per 3½ ounces. It has more than double the calcium of the equivalent amount of milk. And it has other important nutrients for the bones—magnesium, boron, and vitamin K—that help the body utilize calcium. When you think about keeping your bones young and strong, think kale.

2 cups water
1 pound kale, chopped
2 tablespoons extra-virgin olive oil
2 tablespoons finely chopped yellow onion

2 garlic cloves, minced
½ teaspoon sea salt or Celtic salt
½ teaspoon freshly ground black pepper
¼ teaspoon crushed red pepper

1. Bring the water to a boil in a large stockpot or Dutch oven. Add the kale, cover, and cook 2 minutes or until the kale is bright green and wilted. Drain the kale in a colander and press until barely moist.
2. Add the oil to a large skillet and sauté the onion and garlic over low heat for 4 to 5 minutes. Stir in the kale, salt, black pepper, and red pepper. Increase the heat to medium-high and cook for 3 to 4 minutes, stirring constantly. Serve hot.

Makes 6 servings

Nutritional analysis (per serving): 81 calories (51% from fat) • 5g fat • 3g protein • 8g carbohydrate • 2g dietary fiber • 0mg cholesterol • 213mg sodium

Gingered Beets with Sesame

This dish makes a nice warm side dish or a cold salad. Beets are rich in iron and beta-carotene.

4 beets with greens, scrubbed, trimmed, and diced, and the greens chopped
1 tablespoon light soy sauce or tamari
1 tablespoon extra-virgin olive oil

1 tablespoon minced fresh ginger root
½ cup grated carrots
2 teaspoons toasted sesame seeds

1. In a medium saucepan over medium-high heat, boil or steam the beets until tender, 30 to 40 minutes.
2. Steam the greens until wilted, 3 to 4 minutes.
3. In a medium bowl, whisk together the soy sauce or tamari, olive oil, and ginger.
4. Add the beets, greens, carrot, and sesame seeds and toss.
5. Serve warm as a side dish or cold as a side salad.

   Makes 4 servings

Nutritional analysis (per serving): 105 calories (46% from fat) • 6g fat • 3g protein • 12g carbohydrate • 4.5g dietary fiber • 0mg cholesterol • 350mg sodium

Mediterranean Rice Pilaf

~~~~~~

This rice pilaf works both as a side dish and as a stuffing. Abundant in the mineral manganese, this dish provides almost 2 milligrams—the recommended daily amount is 2.5 to 5 milligrams, with the optimum being 15 to 30 milligrams a day. Manganese is a component of the enzyme superoxide dismutase (SOD), which prevents free radical damage implicated in degeneration of tissue associated with the aging process.

1 tablespoon virgin coconut oil
½ cup pine nuts
1 large white or yellow onion, chopped
4 large garlic cloves, minced
1 tablespoon chopped fresh basil or 1 teaspoon dried basil
1 teaspoon dried oregano
Sea salt or Celtic salt and freshly ground black pepper to taste

1 cup long grain brown rice
3 cups vegetable or chicken stock or water
2 vegetable bouillon cubes
1 tablespoon fresh lemon juice
1 teaspoon finely chopped lemon peel

1. Preheat oven to 375°F.
2. Heat the oil in a medium skillet over medium-low heat and sauté the pine nuts for 3 minutes. Add the onion, garlic, basil, oregano, salt, and pepper and cook for 5 minutes. Add the rice, stir well, and cook for 1 minute. Add the stock, bouillon, lemon juice, and peel or zest and bring to a boil, then remove from the stove.
3. Transfer the mixture to an oiled 1½ quart casserole dish and bake for 45 minutes to 1 hour, or until all the liquid is absorbed.

Makes 6 servings

Nutritional analysis (per serving): 210 calories (37% from fat) • 9g fat • 5.5g protein • 28g carbohydrate • 2g dietary fiber • 0mg cholesterol • 207mg sodium

BREADS AND MUFFINS

Blue Cornmeal Muffins

Blue cornmeal is higher in protein and sweeter than yellow cornmeal, making it desirable for baked goods.

1 cup blue cornmeal
1 cup barley flour
4 teaspoons aluminum-free
   baking powder
1 teaspoon sea salt or Celtic salt
1 cup dairy, almond, or rice milk

1 egg, slightly beaten
¼ cup pure maple syrup or birch
   sugar (xylitol)
¼ cup virgin coconut oil or
   butter (melted if solid)

1. Preheat the oven to 425°F.
2. In a large bowl, sift together the cornmeal, barley flour, baking powder, and salt.
3. In a small bowl, whisk together the milk, egg, sweetener, and oil or butter.
4. Add the liquid ingredients to the dry ingredients, stirring just until moistened. Pour the batter into 12 oiled and floured muffin cups (or use paper cup liners), filling each about ¾ full.
5. Bake the muffins until a toothpick inserted into the center of a muffin comes out clean, about 20 to 25 minutes. Remove from the oven and allow to cool on a wire rack for about 10 minutes.
   Makes 12 muffins

Nutritional analysis (per muffin): 121 calories (11% from fat) • 2g fat • 3g protein •
24g carbohydrate • 2g dietary fiber • 18mg cholesterol • 356mg sodium

Savory Rosemary-Onion Muffins

~~~~~

These fragrant muffins transform a soup or salad into a richly satisfying meal. The rosemary is stimulating to the digestive system and is good for the liver and gallbladder. It also is known to improve circulation and strengthen fragile blood vessels, which is particularly important if you tend to bruise easily.

½ to ¾ cup finely chopped yellow onion
1 tablespoon virgin coconut oil
1 egg
1 cup dairy, almond, or rice milk
¼ cup plain yogurt
1 cup coarsely chopped cheddar cheese
2 tablespoons finely minced fresh parsley
1 cup whole wheat pastry flour
½ cup barley flour
½ cup rolled oats (not instant)
2 teaspoons aluminum-free baking powder
2 teaspoons chopped fresh rosemary or 1 teaspoon dried rosemary
1 teaspoon sea salt or Celtic salt
½ teaspoon baking soda
½ teaspoon dry mustard

1. Preheat the oven to 375°F.
2. In a small skillet over low heat, sauté the onion in coconut oil until translucent, about 5 minutes. Set aside and allow the onions to cool.
3. In a small bowl, beat the egg and whisk in the milk and yogurt. Stir in the cheese and parsley; then add the cooled onion.
4. In a large bowl, sift together the pastry flour and barley flour. Stir in the remaining ingredients.
5. Fold the liquid ingredients into the dry ingredients just until mixed. Pour the batter into 12 oiled and floured muffin cups or use paper cup liners, filling each about ¾ full.

6. Bake the muffins until a toothpick inserted into the center of a muffin comes out clean, about 20 to 25 minutes. Remove from the oven and allow to cool on a wire rack for about 10 minutes.
   Makes 12 muffins

Nutritional analysis (per muffin): 72 calories (21% from fat) • 2g fat • 3g protein • 12g carbohydrate • 2g dietary fiber • 19mg cholesterol • 507mg sodium

DESSERTS

Fresh Strawberries with Coconut Sauce

You can substitute other fresh berries for the strawberries.

- ½ cup coconut milk
- 1 tablespoon pure maple syrup or equivalent of healthy low-carb sweetener
- ½ teaspoon pure vanilla extract
- 2 pints fresh strawberries, hulled and quartered
- ¼ cup dried unsweetened coconut flakes, toasted

1. Heat the coconut milk in a small saucepan until almost boiling. Remove from the heat.
2. Whisk in the maple syrup and vanilla.

3. Divide the strawberries among 4 dessert bowls or tall parfait glasses. Drizzle with the coconut sauce and sprinkle a tablespoon of coconut flakes on top.

Makes 4 servings

Nutritional analysis (per serving): 150 calories (52% from fat) • 9g fat • 2g protein • 18g carbohydrate • 4g dietary fiber • 0mg cholesterol • 18mg sodium

Fresh Strawberry Pie with Coconut Crust

This has to be one of the world's healthiest strawberry pies. Strawberries have a high vitamin C content—higher than oranges and orange juice—and they're a low-sugar fruit.

Coconut Piecrust

¾ cup whole wheat pastry flour
½ cup rolled oats (not instant)
½ cup finely shredded unsweetened coconut
¼ cup virgin coconut oil (melted if solid)
2 tablespoons water, as needed

1½ to 2 pints fresh strawberries, hulled, sliced, and chilled
1 cup water
1 heaping tablespoon agar flakes*
¼ cup pure maple syrup

To make the piecrust:

1. Preheat the oven to 375°F.
2. Place the flour, oats, and coconut in a small bowl and mix well. Stir in the oil and gradually add water until the mixture holds together when pressed.

3. Transfer the mixture to a 9-inch pie pan and press against the sides and bottom of the pan. Poke several holes in the sides and bottom of the crust with a fork.

4. Bake for 20 minutes or until the crust is golden brown. Set aside to cool.

To make the pie:

5. Fill the cooled piecrust with sliced strawberries, reserving 1 cup of strawberries, and place in the refrigerator.

6. In a small saucepan, combine the water and agar flakes. Add the cup of strawberries. Bring the mixture to a boil. Reduce the heat and simmer for about 10 minutes, or until the agar is completely dissolved.

7. Place the strawberry-agar mixture in a blender, add the maple syrup, and blend until smooth. Pour this mixture in a small bowl and place in the refrigerator to let it cool for about 15 minutes, or just until it starts jelling. (Make sure the mixture isn't poured into the piecrust hot or it will cause it to turn soggy.)

8. Pour the cooled strawberry-agar mixture over the strawberries in the piecrust and chill for about 2 hours before serving.

*Agar flakes can be found at most health food stores.
   Makes 8 servings

Nutritional analysis (per serving): 180 calories (49% from fat) • 11g fat • 2.5g protein • 22g carbohydrate • 3.5g dietary fiber • 0mg cholesterol • 4.5mg sodium

Acknowledgments

I wish to express my deep and lasting appreciation to all the people who have assisted me with this book, especially my editor, Kristen Jennings, whose creative input totally transformed this book. A very special thanks goes to my literary agent, Pamela Harty, whose friendship and professional expertise is invaluable. You are one of God's gifts to me, and I'm so glad I found you. To John, my husband—you're such great support, my best friend, and a very blessed gift. And most of all to God, who answered many prayers concerning this project, I offer my eternal gratitude.

Appendix A
Cooking Grains

GRAIN (1 cup dry measure)	LIQUID	COOKING TIME	YIELD
Amaranth	2 cups	30 minutes	2 cups
Barley	2 cups	60 minutes	4 cups
Buckwheat	1 to 1½ cups	20 minutes	3½ cups
Bulgur (parboiled, cracked wheat)	1½ cups	15 minutes	2½ cups
Cornmeal (coarse polenta)	3 to 4 cups	25 minutes	2 cups
Cracked wheat	1½ cups	25 minutes	2½ cups
Kamut	1½ cups	1½ hours	2 cups
Millet	2 to 2½ cups	15 to 20 minutes	4 cups

Oats
  rolled
  steel-cut
  whole groats
	
	2 cups
	2 cups
	2 cups
		
		10 minutes
		15 to 20 minutes
		60 minutes
			
			3 cups
			3 cups
			3 cups

Quinoa	2 cups	10 to 15 minutes	2 to 2¼ cups
Rice (all varieties)	1½ to 1¾ cups	45 to 50 minutes	2 cups
Spelt	1¼ to 1½ cups	1 to 1¼ hours	2 cups
Triticale	1¾ cups	2 hours	2½ cups
Wheat berries	1½ cups	2 hours	2½ cups
Wild rice	1¾ cups	55 to 60 minutes	2½ cups

Appendix B
Questionnaires and a Quiz

HOW INSULIN RESISTANT ARE YOU?

PART 1

1. Do you spend more time than you'd like to worrying about your weight? (Score 1 for yes, 0 for no.) _____

2. Do you feel sleepy or fatigued an hour or two after eating? (Score 1 for yes, 0 for no.) _____

3. Do you experience anxiety or panic attacks? (Score 1 for yes, 0 for no.) _____

4. Score 1 point for every symptom you have from the list below:

   Abnormal triglycerides or cholesterol levels _____

   Binge eating, uncontrollable cravings _____

   Bloating or abdominal gas _____

   Chronic fatigue _____

   Chronic indigestion _____

   Depression that comes and goes _____

   Food/chemical allergies _____

Gastrointestinal (digestive tract) problems   _____

Heart trouble (heart attack, congestive heart
failure, etc.)   _____

Hypertension (high blood pressure)   _____

Inability to lose weight on a low-fat diet   _____

Infertility/irregular menstrual periods   _____

Mental confusion or "brain fog"   _____

Obesity (20 percent or more over your ideal weight)   _____

                                           Total Part 1   _____

PART 2

1. Measure your waist and hips. Divide your waist
   measurement by your hip measurement.

   Women: If the result is 0.8 or more, score 10 points   _____

   Men: If the result is 1.0 or more, score 10 points   _____

2. Give yourself one point for every blood relative
   who has diabetes.   _____

3. By how many pounds are you overweight?   _____

4. Give yourself 1 point for every time you've gone on a diet.   _____

                                           Total Part 2   _____
                                 Total Parts 1 and 2   _____

Interpreting the results

Part 1: The maximum possible score is 20. The higher your score, the
greater the likelihood that you will benefit from the lifestyle changes outlined in this book.

Part 2: There is no maximum score. If you recorded a 10 in answer to the first question, you are by definition insulin resistant. If you scored the first question as 0 but your total in part 2 is 15 or more, you have reason to be concerned.

A total for both parts of 35 or more tells you it's time to take action.

This test is taken from *Blood Sugar Blues*, Miryam Ehrlich Williamson.

CANDIDA QUESTIONNAIRE

If you suspect you might suffer from candidiasis, W. G. Crook, MD, has developed a questionnaire that you can fill out to determine the likelihood. There are different point scores for each question. Note the points and add them up. The score evaluation is at the end of the quiz.

I. HISTORY	POINT SCORE
1. Have you taken tetracycline or other antibiotics for acne for one month or longer?	25
2. Have you at any time in your life taken other "broad-spectrum" antibiotics for respiratory, urinary, or other infections for two months or longer, or in short courses four or more times in a one-year period?	20
3. Have you ever taken a broad-spectrum antibiotic (even a single course)?	6
4. Have you at any time in your life been bothered by persistent prostatitis, vaginitis, or other problems affecting your reproductive organs?	25

5. Have you been pregnant one time?	3
Two or more times?	5
6. Have you taken birth-control pills for six months to two years?	8
For more than two years?	15
7. Have you taken prednisone or other cortisone-type drugs for two weeks or less?	6
For more than two weeks?	15
8. Does exposure to perfumes, insecticides, fabric shop odors, and other chemicals provoke mild symptoms?	5
Moderate to severe symptoms?	20
9. Are your symptoms worse on damp, muggy days or in moldy places?	20
10. Have you had athlete's foot, ringworm, "jock itch," or other chronic infections of the skin or nails?	
Mild to moderate?	10
Severe or persistent?	20
11. Do you crave sugar?	10
12. Do you crave breads?	10
13. Do you crave alcoholic beverages?	10
14. Does tobacco smoke really bother you?	10

Total Score for This Section _____

II. Major Symptoms   Point Score

For each of your symptoms below, enter the appropriate figure in the Point Score Column.

If symptom is occasional or mild	score 3 points
If symptom is frequent and/or moderately severe	score 6 points
If symptom is severe and/or disabling	score 9 points

1. Fatigue or lethargy   _____

2. Feeling of being drained   _____

3. Poor memory   _____

4. Feeling "spacey" or "unreal"   _____

5. Depression   _____

6. Numbness, burning, or tingling   _____

7. Muscle aches   _____

8. Muscle weakness or paralysis   _____

9. Pain and/or swelling in joints   _____

10. Abdominal pain   _____

11. Constipation   _____

12. Diarrhea   _____

13. Bloating   _____

14. Persistent vaginal itch   _____

15. Persistent vaginal burning   _____

16. Prostatitis   _____

17. Impotence   _____

18. Loss of sexual desire   _____

19. Endometriosis   _____

20. Cramping and other menstrual irregularities   _____

21. Premenstrual tension   _____

22. Spots in front of eyes   _____

23. Erratic vision   _____

Total Score for This Section   _____

III. OTHER SYMPTOMS

For each of the symptoms below, enter the appropriate figure in the Point Score Column.

If symptom is occasional or mild   score 1 point

If symptom is frequent and/or moderately severe   score 2 points

If symptom is severe and/or disabling   score 3 points

1. Drowsiness   _____

2. Irritability   _____

3. Lack of coordination   _____

4. Inability to concentrate   _____

5. Frequent mood swings   _____

6. Headache   _____

7. Dizziness/loss of balance   _____

8. Pressure above ears, feeling of head swelling and tingling   _____

9. Itching   _____

10. Other rashes   _____

11. Heartburn   _____

12. Indigestion   _____

13. Belching and intestinal gas   _____

14. Mucus in stools   _____

15. Hemorrhoids   _____

16. Dry mouth   _____

17. Rash or blisters in mouth   _____

18. Bad breath   _____

19. Joint swelling or arthritis   _____

20. Nasal congestion or discharge   _____

21. Postnasal drip   _____

22. Nasal itching   _____

23. Sore or dry throat   _____

24. Cough   _____

25. Pain or tightness in chest   _____

26. Wheezing or shortness of breath   _____

27. Urinary urgency or frequency   _____

28. Burning on urination   _____

29. Failing vision   _____

30. Burning or tearing of eyes   _____

31. Recurrent infections or fluid in ears   _____

32. Ear pain or deafness   _____

Total Score for This Section   _____

Total score from Section I   _____

Total score from Section II   _____

Total score from Section III   _____

Total All Sections   _____

	WOMEN	MEN
Yeast-connected health problems are almost certainly present	>180	>140
Yeast-connected health problems are probably present	120–180	90–140
Yeast-connected health problems are possibly present	60–119	40–89
Yeast-connected health problems are less likely to be present	<60	<40

This questionnaire is adapted from W. G. Crook, *The Yeast Connection.*

Although the Candida Questionnaire can help determine your condition, ultimately the best method for diagnosing candidiasis is clinical evaluation by a physician knowledgeable about yeast-related illness.

THYROID HEALTH QUIZ
(SYMPTOMS OF AN UNDERACTIVE THYROID)

Score 1 point for each symptom that applies to you.

_____ Appetite problems, severely reduced or excessive

_____ Bloating or indigestion after eating

_____ Low body temperature (below 97.6°F, resting)

_____ Weight gain

_____ Mucus accumulation

_____ Hoarse throat

_____ Cold hands and feet

_____ Puffy eyes

_____ Constipation

_____ Decreased sweating

_____ Dry mouth (drinking water doesn't help much)

_____ Intolerance to cold or heat

_____ Poor digestion of animal products

_____ Poor absorption of minerals

_____ Sluggish lymph drainage

_____ Swelling (ankles, eyelids, face, feet, hands, lymph nodes, throat)

_____ Spleen or liver problems

_____ Calcium deficiency

_____ Carpal tunnel syndrome

_____ Left arm weakness

_____ Muscle/joint problems (knees, elbows, etc.)

_____ Numbness in fingers

_____ Stiff neck

_____ Tenderness in lower ribs

_____ Brittle nails

_____ Grooves or ridges in nails

_____ Thin, peeling nails

_____ Slow-growing nails

_____ White spots on nails (this can also be a zinc deficiency)

_____ Fluttering in ears

_____ Occasional stinging in eyes

_____ Poor vision

_____ Impotency

_____ Loss of libido/low sex drive

_____ Miscarriages

_____ Premature deliveries

_____ Spontaneous abortions

_____ Stillbirths

_____ Coarse, dry hair

_____ Hair loss

_____ Loss of hair on arms, underarms, legs, eyebrows, scalp

_____ Elevated cholesterol

_____ Enlargement of heart

_____ Heart pain

_____ Hypertension

_____ Pain in diaphragm

_____ Heart palpitations

_____ Impaired heart function

_____ Slower heart rate

_____ Sense of pressure (compression) on chest

_____ PMS

_____ Prolonged or heavy menstrual bleeding

_____ Light menstrual flow

_____ Shorter menstrual cycle

_____ Bipolarity (manic-depression)

_____ Depression

_____ Difficulty concentrating

_____ Emotional instability

_____ Fatigue/lack of energy

_____ Forgetfulness

_____ Inability to "drag oneself from bed"

_____ Lethargy

_____ Nervousness

_____ Restlessness

_____ Shyness

_____ Tendency to cry easily

_____ Chronic mucus in head/nose (thyroid governs mucus production)

_____ Shortness of breath

_____ Difficulty drawing deep breath

_____ Gasping for air occasionally

_____ Intolerance to closed, stuffy rooms

_____ Loss of smell

_____ Need for fresh air

_____ Sleep disturbances

_____ Grinding teeth during sleep

_____ Loss of hearing

A score of 20 points or more may be indicative of low thyroid. Although the Thyroid Quiz can help you determine your thyroid health, ultimately the best method for diagnosis is clinical evaluation by a physician knowledgeable in thyroid health. I recommend you see a physician who can treat your condition holistically.

References

CHAPTER 1 · WHAT CAUSES WRINKLES?

Anderson, Richard, ND. *Cleanse and Purify Thyself Book 1.5* (Mt. Shasta, CA: Triumph, 1998), 14–326.

Blaylock, Russell L., MD. *Excitotoxins: The Taste That Kills* (Santa Fe, NM: Health Press, 1997).

Bueno-Aguer, Lee. *Fast Your Way to Health* (New Kensington, PA: Whitaker House, 1991), 117–22.

Bracciante, Lara Evans. "Time Is on Your Side: Antiaging Secrets." *Taste for Life* (September 2003), 53–56.

Calbom, Cherie, MS. "Thyroid Health: A Key to Weight Loss." www.mercola.com/2003/nov/8 (November 8, 2003).

"Chronic Fatigue Syndrome May Be Linked to Hormonal Deficiency." *Infectious Disease News* (February 1992), 1, 4.

Eliot, Robert S. "Stress and the Heart: Mechanisms, Measurement, and Management." *Postgraduate Medicine* 92 (5) (October 1992): 237–48.

"Erogenic Nutrients, Nonnutrients, and Drugs." *Equine Veterinary Data* 13 (6) (1992): 271.

Kovalovich, Lisa. "Can You Reverse Sun Damage?" *Ladies Home Journal*. www.lhj.com/lhj/story; html?storyid-/templatedata/lhj/story.data/CanYouReverseSunDamage_05132004.xml.

Naylor, Mark F., MD, and Kevin C. Farmer. "Sun Damage and Prevention." www.telemedicine.org/stamford.html.

Perricone, Nicholas, MD. *The Perricone Prescription* (New York: Warner, 2002).

Rosedale, Ron, MD. "Insulin and Its Metabolic Effects." www.mercola.com/2001/jul/14/insulin.htm.

Schedlowski, Manfred, et al. "Acute Psychological Stress Increases Plasma Levels of Cortisol, Prolactin, and TSH." *Life Sciences* 50 (1992): 1201–05.

"Skin Cancer: Saving Your Skin from Sun Damage." familydoctor.org/x5152/xml.

Whitaker, Julian, MD. "Smile and Get Well." *Health & Healing* 13, 8 (August 2003), 1–2.

Yin, D. "Is Carbonyl Detoxification an Important Aspect of the Aging Process During Sleep?" *Medical Hypotheses* 54 (4) (April 2000): 519–22.

CHAPTER 2 • THE WRINKLE CLEANSE FOODS

Batmanghelidj, F., MD. *Your Body's Many Cries for Water* (Falls Church, VA: Global Health Solutions, 1995).

Bracciante, Lara Evans. "Time Is on Your Side: Antiaging Secrets." *Taste for Life* (September 2003), 53–56.

Bueno-Aguer, Lee. *Fast Your Way to Health* (New Kensington, PA: Whitaker House, 1991).

Calbom, Cherie. *The Coconut Diet* (New York: Warner Books, 2005).

Clement, Brian R., with Theresa Foy DiGeronimo. *Living Foods for Optimum Health* (Rocklin, CA: Prima Publishing, 1996), 163–68.

Fallon, Sally. *Nourishing Traditions* (San Diego: ProMotion Publishing, 1995), 9.

Goldbeck, Nikki, and David Goldbeck. *The Goldbecks' Guide to Good Food* (New York: New American Library, 1987).

Kenton, Leslie, and Susannah Kenton. *Raw Energy* (London: Century Publishing, 1984), 109–110.

Krause, Marie V., and L. Kathleen Mahan. *Food, Nutrition & Diet Therapy,* 7th Ed. (Philadelphia: W.B. Saunders Company, 1984).

Lieberman, Shari, and Nancy Bruning. *The Real Vitamin & Mineral Book* (New York: Avery, 1990).

Mabey, Richard. *The New Age Herbalist* (New York: Collier Books, 1988).

Murray, Michael T., ND. *Encyclopedia of Nutritional Supplements* (Rocklin, CA: Prima Publishing, 1996).

Perricone, Nicholas, MD. *The Perricone Prescription* (New York: Harper Resource, 2002).

Purba, M. Kouris-Blazos, et al. "Skin Wrinkling: Can Food Make a Difference?" *Journal of the American College of Nutrition* 20 (1) (2001): 71–80.

Rosedale, Ron, MD. "Insulin and Its Metabolic Effects." Paper presented at Designs for Health Institute's BoulderFest, August 1999 Seminar. www.mercola.com/2001/jul/14/insulin.htm., 6.

Sison, A. "Blueberries May Reverse Some Aging." *Medical Tribune* 40 (17) (October 1999): 4.

Trichopoulous, A., and E. Vasilopoulous. "Mediterranean Diet and Longevity." *British Journal of Nutrition* 84 (Suppl. 2) (2000): S205–209.

Wigmore, Ann. *The Wheatgrass Book* (New York: Avery Publishing, 1985).

Worthington, Virginia. "Nutritional Quality of Organic Versus Conventional Fruits, Vegetables and Grains," *Journal of Alternative and Complementary Medicine* 7 (2) (2001):161–73.

CHAPTER 3 • SUBSTANCES THAT ACCELERATE AGING

"Aspartame and Dieting." *Nutrition Week* 27 (23) (June 13, 1997); *International Journal of Obesity* 21 (1) (January 1997): 37–42.

Calbom, Cherie. *The Coconut Diet* (New York: Warner Books, 2005).

Enig, Mary G. *Know Your Fats* (Silver Springs, MD: Bethesda Press, 2000).

Fallon, Sally. *Nourishing Traditions* (San Diego: ProMotion Publishing, 1995).

Goldbeck, Nikki, and David Goldbeck. *The Goldbecks' Guide to Good Food* (New York: New American Library, 1987).

Lieberman, Shari, and Nancy Bruning. *The Real Vitamin & Mineral Book* (New York: Avery, 1990).

Mercola, Joseph. "The Potential Dangers of Sucralose." www.mercola.com/2000/dec/3/sucralose_dangers.htm

Perricone, Nicholas, MD. *The Perricone Prescription* (New York: Harper Resource, 2002).

Purba, M. Kouris-Blazos, et al. "Skin Wrinkling: Can Food Make a Difference?" *Journal of the American College of Nutrition* 20 (1) (2001): 71–80.

Roberts, H. J. "Does Aspartame Cause Human Brain Cancer?" *Journal of Advancement in Medicine.* 4 (4) (winter 1991): 231–41.

Rosedale, Ron, MD. "Insulin and Its Metabolic Effects." Paper presented at Designs for Health Institute's BoulderFest, August 1999 Seminar. www.mercola.com/2001/jul/14/insulin.htm., 6.

Wesley-Hosford, Zia. *The Beautiful Body Book* (New York: Bantam, 1984).

CHAPTER 4 • STEP 1: THE QUICK START PROGRAMS

Haas, Elson M., MD. "Nutritional Program for Fasting." www.healthy.net/scr/article.asp?

Walker, N. W., DSc. *Become Younger* (Prescott, AZ: Norwalk Press, 1978).

CHAPTER 5 • STEP 2: THE 14-DAY WRINKLE CLEANSE DIET

Barzilai, N., and G. Gupta. "Revisiting the Role of Fat Mass in the Life Extension Induced by Caloric Restriction." *The Journals of Gerontology. Series A, Biological Sciences and Medical Sciences* 54 (1999): B89–96.

Chung, Hy, J. H. Kim, et al. "Molecular Inflammation Hypothesis of Aging Based on the Anti-aging Mechanism of Calorie Restriction." *Microscopy Research and Technique* 59 (4) (November 15, 2002): 264–72.

Kemnitz, J. W., et al. "Dietary Restriction Increases Insulin Sensitivity and Lowers Blood Glucose in Rhesus Monkeys." *American Journal of Physiology* 256 (1994): E540–47.

Lane, M.A., et al. "Diet Restriction in Rhesus Monkeys Lowers Fasting and Glucose-stimulated Glucoregulatory End Points." *American Journal of Physiology* 268 (1995): E941–48.

Lass, A., et al. "Caloric Restriction Prevents Age-associated Accrual of Oxidative Damage to Mouse Skeletal Muscle Mitochondria." *Free Radical Biology & Medicine* 25 (1998): 1089–97.

Masoro, E. J. "Possible Mechanisms Underlying the Antiaging Actions of Caloric Restriction." *Toxicologic Pathology* 24 (1996): 738–41.

Masoro, E. J., and S. N. Austad. "The Evolution of the Antiaging Action of Dietary Restriction: A Hypothesis." *The Journals of Gerontology. Series A, Biological Sciences and Medical Sciences* 51 (1996): B387–91.

Masoro, E. J., et al. "Dietary Restriction Alters Characteristics of Glucose Fuel Use." *Journal of Gerontology* 47 (1992): B202–208.

Mattison, J. A., et al. "Calorie Restriction in Rhesus Monkeys." *Experimental Gerontology* 38 (2003): 35–46.

Roth, G.S., et al. "Biomarkers of Caloric Restriction May Predict Longevity in Humans." *Science* 297 (2002): 811.

Taubes, G. "The Famine of Youth." *Scientific American Presents* 11 (2000): 44–49.

Van Remmen, H., Z. Guo, and A. Richardson. "The Anti-aging Action of Dietary Restriction." *Novartis Foundation Symposium* 235 (2001): 221–33.

Wang, Z. Q., et al. "Effect of Age and Caloric Restriction on Insulin Receptor Binding and Glucose Transporter Levels in Aging Rats." *Experimental Gerontology* 32 (1997): 671–84.

Weindruch, R., and R. L. Walford. *The Retardation of Aging and Disease by Dietary Restriction.* (Springfield, IL: Thomas, 1988), 7–215.

Weindruch, R., et al. "The Retardation of Aging in Mice by Dietary Restriction: Longevity, Cancer, Immunity and Lifetime Energy Intake." *Journal of Nutrition* 116 (1986): 641–54.

CHAPTER 6 • STEP 3: THE CLEANSING BOOST PROGRAMS

Anderson, Richard, ND. *Cleanse & Purify Thyself* (Mt. Shasta, CA: Triumph, 1998), 277, 299, 300, 307, 310.

———. *The Liver* (Mt. Shasta, CA: Triumph, 1999).

Cabot, Sandra, MD. *The Liver Cleansing Diet* (Scottsdale, AZ: SBC International, 1996).

Frahm, David. "Feed Your Thyroid." *Health Quarters Monthly* (September 2004).

"Internal Autumn Cleanse." *Healing Lifestyles & Spas* (September–October 2004), 46–50.

Jensen, Bernard. *Dr. Jensen's Guide to Better Bowel Health* (New York: Avery, 1999).

Page, Linda. *Detoxification* (Carmel Valley, CA: Healthy Healing Publications, 1999).

Walker, Shanagh. *Cellulite: Not Just a Fancy Name for Fat* (Sydney: Harper Collins, 2001), 42–43.

CHAPTER 7 • STEP 4: VITAMINS AND MINERALS THAT FIGHT AGING

Engstrom, James E. "Vitamin C Intake and Mortality Among a Sample of the United States Population." *Epidemiology* 3 (3) (May 1992): 195–202.

Henson, D. E,. et al. "Does Vitamin C Protect Against UVA and UVB?" *Patient Care* 83 (May 30, 1992): 547–50.

Jayachandran, M., et al. "Status of Lipids, Lipid Peroxidation, and Antioxidant Systems with Vitamin C Supplementation during Aging Rats." *Journal of Nutritional Biochemistry* 7 (1996): 270–75.

Lassus, A. "Colloidal Silicic Acid for Oral and Topical Treatment of Aged Skin, Fragile Hair, and Brittle Nails in Females." *Journal of International Medical Research* 21 (1993): 209–15.

Malik, Nageena S., and Keith M. Meek. "Vitamins and Analgesics in the Prevention of Collagen Ageing," *Age and Ageing* 25 (1996): 279–84.

Murray, Michael T. *Encyclopedia of Nutritional Supplements* (Rocklin, CA: Prima Publishing, 1996), 229–23, 296–97, 343–46.

Perricone, Nicholas, MD. *The Wrinkle Cure* (New York: Warner Books, 2000), 67–80.

Sinatra, Stephen, MD. "Bone Health Program." *The Sinatra Health Report* (August 2004), 5.

Whitaker, Julian. *Health & Healing* 12 (6) (June 2002): 3.

———. *Health & Healing* 14 (6) (June 2004): 5.

Resources

CHERIE CALBOM'S WEBSITES

www.wrinklecleanse.com

www.gococonuts.com, Information on *The Coconut Diet: The Secret Ingredient That Helps You Lose Weight While Eating Your Favorite Foods* (New York: Warner Books, 2005).

OTHER WEBSITES FOR CHERIE CALBOM

www.juicinginfo.com, www.cleansinginfo.com, www.ultimatesmoothie.com, and www.cancercleanse.com

PRODUCTS

COCONUT PRODUCTS

Organic virgin coconut oil: 1-866-8GET-WEL

FREE RADICAL TEST KIT

The free radical monitor is a simple-to-use home urine test that you can use to assess the activity of free radicals in the body.

Free radical monitor: The Home Antioxidant Test, 1-800-923-8935

OTHER FOOD PRODUCTS

Cod Liver Oil

Olde World Icelandic Cod Liver Oil: Garden of Life, www.gardenoflifeusa.com; 800-622-8986

Carlson's Cod Liver Oil: www.mercola.com/forms/carlsons.htm (Can be found at most health food stores.)

Sugar

Pure birch sugar: The Ultimate Sweetener, 1-800-843-6325

PHASE II CLEANSE PRODUCTS

Colon Cleanse

Fiber Max, Colon Cleanse I and II: Advanced Naturals (Can be found at health foods stores.)

Psyllium, bentonite, herbal nutrition, and chomper: Arise & Shine Products, 1-866-8GETWEL

Super Seed—fiber only: Garden of Life, www.gardenoflifeusa.com; 1-800-622-8986

Liver Cleanse

Liver Life I and II: Arise & Shine, 1-866-8GETWEL

Liver Cleanse: Thorne, 1-866-8GETWEL

Gallbladder Cleanse

Lipo-Gen: Metagenics, 1-866-8GETWEL

Kidney Cleanse Herbs

Kidney Life: Arise & Shine, 1-866-8GETWEL

Candida albicans Cleanse Products

Fungal Defense: Garden of Life, www.gardenoflifeusa.com; 1-800-622-8986

Candida Cleanse: Silver Creek Labs, 1-800-493-1146

Yeast Max: Advanced Naturals (Can be found at health food stores.)

Parasite Cleanse Products

ParaCleanse: Silver Creek Labs, 1-800-493-1146

Worm Squirm I and II: Arise & Shine, 1-866-8GETWEL

SUPPLEMENTS AND RELATED PRODUCTS

Enzymes

Digest chewables by Ness Formula (natural raspberry-flavored chewables that provide a full spectrum of enzymes with silica): 1-866-8GETWEL

Goat Protein

Goatein: Garden of Life, www.gardenoflifeusa.com; 1-800-622-8986

Juice Concentrates

(All juice concentrates can be found at most health food stores.)

Black cherry juice concentrate: Dynamic Health

Cranberry juice concentrate: Dynamic Health

Elderberry juice concentrate: Natural Sources

Thyroid and Adrenal Support

Adrenal support: Androgen—Metagenics, 1-866-8GETWEL

Liquid iodine: Biotics Research, 1-866-8GETWEL

Thyroid support: Thyrosol—Metagenics, 1-866-8GETWEL

Minerals

Bio-available liquid minerals: Eniva Essentials, 1-866-8GETWEL

Probiotics

Primal Defense: Garden of Life, www.gardenoflifeusa.com; 1-800-622-8986

Ultra Flora Plus DF Capsules: Metagenics, 1-866-8GETWEL

Sleep Aids

Tranquilnite: New Chapter (Can be found at health food stores.)

Melatonin: Source Naturals (Can be found at health food stores.)

SKIN CARE

Coconut cream—moisturizing cream and lotion: Tropical Traditions, 1-866-311-COCO

Epicuren Basic Home Care Kit (the famous enzyme facial): 1-800-779-0088

EPIONCE PRODUCTS: 1-800-923-8935

Renewal Eye Cream:
Stimulates skin renewal, improves firmness and elasticity, diminishes the appearance of fine lines, wrinkles, puffiness, dark circles, and uneven skin tone

Renewal Facial Lotion:
Designed to reverse the visible signs of aging while preventing future skin damage

Lytic Lotion:
Cleans pores, removes skin scales, and reduces redness; also eliminates bumps, blackheads, whiteheads, and other bumps. Lytic Lotion used with Renewal Facial Lotion helps to reverse actinic keratosis, which can lead to skin cancer.

EMINENCE (HANDMADE ORGANIC SKIN CARE FROM HUNGARY): 1-800-923-8935

Cleanser: Lemon cleanser (all skin types); Sweet Red Rose cleanser (sensitive skin)

Toner: Rosehips (oily, acne, rosacea); Red Rose (normal); Wild Plum (dry)

Treatments: AHA Fruit Pulp Treatment with Paprika (exfoliating/stimulating)
   Lime Stimulating Treatment with Mixed Rosehips and Maize Masque
   Almond & Mineral Treatment (exfoliating/stimulating)
   Rosehips & Maize (exfoliating)

Masques (listed from oily to dry skin)
   Herbal Mud
   Menthol Rosehips
   Quince Apple
   Sour Cherry
   Stone Crop
   Sweet Red Rose

Carrot Vitamin

Wild Plum

Pumpkin Orange

Peach

Moisturizers (listed from oily to normal skin)

Thermal Spring Whip

Rosehip Whip

Apricot Whip

Sweet Red Rose Whip

Sour Cherry Whip

Gingko Whip

Wild Plum Whip

Moisturizers (from normal to dry skin)

Stone Crop

Black Perlette Grape

Naseberry Treatment Cream

Linden Calendula Treatment Cream

Rich Black Perlette Grape

Vitamin C (fresh-dried L-ascorbic vitamin C) Serum EC Mode: 1-800-923-8935

Pür Minerals: 1-800-923-8935

Micronized mineral-based products

Powder

Mineral glow

Bronzer

Blush

Eye Shadow

Lipstick

Lipliner

Sunscreen (natural)

UV Natural SP 15 with natural preservatives and vitamins and minerals: 1-800-923-8935

HEALTH CENTERS

The following centers offer a raw foods/juice detoxification program. Most of them offer nutritional classes, and some offer other health classes that address the emotional, mental, and spiritual aspects of health and renewal. Most of the centers also offer massage and colonics. It is best to contact the various centers to find out which one best fits your needs.

Cedar Springs Renewal Center
Michael Mahaffey and Nan Monk, Directors
31459 Barben Road
Sedro Woolley, WA 98284
(360) 826-3599
fax: (360) 422-1524
website: www.cedarsprings.org

HealthQuarters Ministries
David Frahm, ND, Director
3620 W. Colorado Avenue
Colorado Springs, CO 80904
(719) 593-8694
fax: (719) 531-7884
e-mail: healthqu@healthquarters .org
website: healthquarters.org

Hippocrates Institute
Brian and Anna Maria Clement, Directors
1443 Palmdale Ct.
West Palm Beach, FL 33411
(800) 842-2125
fax: (561) 471-9464
e-mail: hippocrates@worldnet.att.net
website: www.hippocratesinstitute.org

Optimum Health Institute of Austin
Route 1, Box 339 J
Cedar Creek, TX 78612
(512) 303-4817
fax: (512) 303-1239
e-mail: austin@optimumhealth.org
website: www.optimumhealth.org

Optimum Health Institute of San Diego
6970 Central Avenue
Lemon Grove, CA 91945-2198
(800) 993-4325
fax: (619) 589-4098
e-mail: optimum@optimumhealth.org
website: www.optimumhealth.org

Sanoviv Medical Institute
Dr. Myron Wentz, Director
2602-C Transportation Avenue
National City, CA 91950
(800) 726-6848
fax: (801) 954-7477
website: www.sanoviv.com

We Care
Susana and Susan Lombardi, Directors
18000 Long Canyon Road
Desert Hot Springs, CA 92241
(800) 888-2523
fax: (760) 251-5399
e-mail: info@wecarespa.com
website: www.wecarespa.com

Index